AN INTEGRATED FRAMEWORK FOR ASSESSING THE VALUE OF COMMUNITY-BASED PREVENTION

Committee on Valuing Community-Based,
Non-Clinical Prevention Policies and Wellness Strategies

Board on Population Health and Public Health Practice

INSTITUTE OF MEDICINE
OF THE NATIONAL ACADEMIES

THE NATIONAL ACADEMIES PRESS
Washington, D.C.
www.nap.edu

THE NATIONAL ACADEMIES PRESS   500 Fifth Street, NW   Washington, DC 20001

NOTICE: The project that is the subject of this report was approved by the Governing Board of the National Research Council, whose members are drawn from the councils of the National Academy of Sciences, the National Academy of Engineering, and the Institute of Medicine. The members of the committee responsible for the report were chosen for their special competences and with regard for appropriate balance.

This study was supported by contracts between the National Academy of Sciences and the California Endowment (20091915), the de Beaumont Foundation, the Robert Wood Johnson Foundation (68317), and the W.K. Kellogg Foundation (P3016629). Any opinions, findings, conclusions, or recommendations expressed in this publication are those of the author(s) and do not necessarily reflect the view of the organizations or agencies that provided support for this project.

International Standard Book Number-13:   978-0-309-26354-2
International Standard Book Number-10:   0-309-26354-9

Additional copies of this report are available from the National Academies Press, 500 Fifth Street, NW, Keck 360, Washington, DC 20001; (800) 624-6242 or (202) 334-3313; http://www.nap.edu.

For more information about the Institute of Medicine, visit the IOM home page at: www.iom.edu.

Suggested citation: IOM (Institute of Medicine). 2012. *An integrated framework for assessing the value of community-based prevention.* Washington, DC: The National Academies Press.

"Knowing is not enough; we must apply. Willing is not enough; we must do."
—Goethe

INSTITUTE OF MEDICINE
OF THE NATIONAL ACADEMIES

Advising the Nation. Improving Health.

THE NATIONAL ACADEMIES
Advisers to the Nation on Science, Engineering, and Medicine

The **National Academy of Sciences** is a private, nonprofit, self-perpetuating society of distinguished scholars engaged in scientific and engineering research, dedicated to the furtherance of science and technology and to their use for the general welfare. Upon the authority of the charter granted to it by the Congress in 1863, the Academy has a mandate that requires it to advise the federal government on scientific and technical matters. Dr. Ralph J. Cicerone is president of the National Academy of Sciences.

The **National Academy of Engineering** was established in 1964, under the charter of the National Academy of Sciences, as a parallel organization of outstanding engineers. It is autonomous in its administration and in the selection of its members, sharing with the National Academy of Sciences the responsibility for advising the federal government. The National Academy of Engineering also sponsors engineering programs aimed at meeting national needs, encourages education and research, and recognizes the superior achievements of engineers. Dr. Charles M. Vest is president of the National Academy of Engineering.

The **Institute of Medicine** was established in 1970 by the National Academy of Sciences to secure the services of eminent members of appropriate professions in the examination of policy matters pertaining to the health of the public. The Institute acts under the responsibility given to the National Academy of Sciences by its congressional charter to be an adviser to the federal government and, upon its own initiative, to identify issues of medical care, research, and education. Dr. Harvey V. Fineberg is president of the Institute of Medicine.

The **National Research Council** was organized by the National Academy of Sciences in 1916 to associate the broad community of science and technology with the Academy's purposes of furthering knowledge and advising the federal government. Functioning in accordance with general policies determined by the Academy, the Council has become the principal operating agency of both the National Academy of Sciences and the National Academy of Engineering in providing services to the government, the public, and the scientific and engineering communities. The Council is administered jointly by both Academies and the Institute of Medicine. Dr. Ralph J. Cicerone and Dr. Charles M. Vest are chair and vice chair, respectively, of the National Research Council.

www.national-academies.org

STEVEN M. TEUTSCH, Chief Science Officer, Los Angeles County Department of Public Health, California
CHAPIN WHITE, Senior Health Researcher, Center for Studying Health System Change, Washington, DC

Consultant

CATHERINE M. JONES, University of Montréal, Canada

Study Staff

LYLA M. HERNANDEZ, Study Director
MELISSA FRENCH, Associate Program Officer
ANDREW LEMERISE, Research Associate
ANGELA MARTIN, Senior Program Assistant
ROSE MARIE MARTINEZ, Director, Board on Population Health and Public Health Practice

Reviewers

This report has been reviewed in draft form by persons chosen for their diverse perspectives and technical expertise, in accordance with procedures approved by the National Research Council's Report Review Committee. The purpose of this independent review is to provide candid and critical comments that will assist the institution in making its published report as sound as possible and to ensure that the report meets institutional standards for objectivity, evidence, and responsiveness to the study charge. The review comments and draft manuscript remain confidential to protect the integrity of the deliberative process. We wish to thank the following individuals for their review of this report:

Laurie M. Anderson, Washington State Institute for Public Policy
Charles C. Branas, University of Pennsylvania
Norman Fost, University of Wisconsin–Madison
Marthe R. Gold, City University of New York Medical School
Dana Goldman, University of Southern California
Mary Mincer Hansen, Des Moines University
Robert Jeffery, University of Minnesota
Michael Maciosek, HealthPartners Research Foundation
Vickie Mays, University of California, Los Angeles
Barbara A. Ormond, The Urban Institute
Patrick Remington, University of Wisconsin–Madison
Barbara Rimer, University of North Carolina

James F. Sallis, University of California, San Diego
Jane E. Sisk, Institute of Medicine
Pierre Vigilance, George Washington University

Although the reviewers listed above have provided many constructive comments and suggestions, they were not asked to endorse the conclusions or recommendations nor did they see the final draft of the report before its release. The review of this report was overseen by **Georges C. Benjamin,** American Public Health Association, and **Charles E. Phelps,** University of Rochester. Appointed by the Institute of Medicine and the National Research Council, they were responsible for making certain that an independent examination of this report was carried out in accordance with institutional procedures and that all review comments were carefully considered. Responsibility for the final content of this report rests entirely with the authoring committee and the institution.

Acknowledgments

Many people contributed to the development of *An Integrated Framework for Assessing the Value of Community-Based Prevention*. The committee would like to acknowledge and thank those individuals whose input invigorated committee deliberations and enhanced the quality of this report.

First, we would like to thank the sponsors of this project, the California Endowment, the de Beaumont Foundation, the Robert Wood Johnson Foundation, and the W.K. Kellogg foundation. We are particularly appreciative of the efforts of Angela McGowan, James Sprague, Marion Standish, and Alice M. Warner-Mehlhorn.

The committee greatly appreciated the input of David Paltiel and Charles Poole and the speakers whose presentations informed committee thinking, including Bridget Booske, Rob Grunewald, Veva Islas-Hooker, M. Rebecca Kilburn, Tyler Norris, Deirdre Oakley, Brian Smedley, Harold Sox, Brenda Spencer, Kenneth Thorpe, Steven H. Woolf, and Chen Zhen.

The committee was very fortunate in its staffing for this study. We wish to thank our study director, Lyla M. Hernandez, and our associate program officer, Melissa French, for their efforts in producing a clearly written, well-organized report that reflects the collective thought of the committee. Our appreciation also goes to Andrew Lemerise for his exceptional research support and tireless efforts in tracking down elusive references, and to Angela Martin for her excellent administrative and logistical support. We were also fortunate that Catharine M. Jones at the University of Montréal was available to provide important research assistance.

Contents

Summary

Over the past century the major causes of morbidity and mortality in the United States have shifted from those related to communicable diseases to those due to chronic diseases. Just as the major causes of morbidity and mortality have changed, so too has understanding of health and what makes people healthy or ill. Research has documented the importance of the social determinants of health (for example, socioeconomic status and education), which affect health directly as well as through their impact on other health determinants such as risk factors. Targeting interventions toward the conditions associated with today's challenges to living a healthy life requires an increased emphasis on the factors that affect the current causes of morbidity and mortality, factors such as the social determinants of health. Many community-based prevention interventions target such conditions.

Community-based prevention interventions offer three distinct strengths. First, because the intervention is implemented population-wide it is inclusive and not dependent on access to the health care system. Second, by directing strategies at an entire population an intervention can reach individuals at all levels of risk. And finally, some lifestyle and behavioral risk factors are shaped by conditions not under an individual's control. For example, encouraging an individual to eat healthy food when none is accessible undermines the potential for successful behavioral change. Community-based prevention interventions can be designed to affect environmental and social conditions that are out of the reach of clinical services.

When a person is ill, making a case for policies and programs to avoid further deterioration of health or death seems reasonable. However, prevention requires that before someone becomes sick, society invest the financial and other resources necessary to make the required changes in individual and community life associated with preventing illness. Some of the persons who receive the intervention would never become sick, yet they share the costs of the intervention. These certain costs of improving health often outweigh the perceived benefits of community-based prevention, especially if individuals perceive their own risk of illness as low.

Four foundations—the California Endowment, the de Beaumont Foundation, the Robert Wood Johnson Foundation, and the W.K. Kellogg Foundation—asked the Institute of Medicine to convene an expert committee to develop a framework for assessing the value of community-based, non-clinical prevention policies and wellness strategies, especially those targeting the prevention of long-term, chronic diseases. The charge to the committee was further defined as follows:

- Define "community-based, non-clinical prevention policy and wellness strategies."
- Define "value" for community-based, non-clinical prevention policy and wellness strategies.
- Analyze current frameworks used to assess the value of community-based, non-clinical prevention policies and wellness strategies, including
    o   the methodologies and measures used and
    o   the short- and long-term impacts of such prevention policy and wellness strategies on communities, including health care spending and public health.
- If warranted, propose a new framework or frameworks that capture the breadth and complexity of community-based, non-clinical prevention policies and wellness strategies, including interventions that target specific behaviors and health outcomes.

The framework should

- consider the sources of data that are needed and available;
- consider the concepts of generalization, scaling up, and sustainability of programs; and
- address national and state policy implications associated with implementing the framework.

DEFINITIONS

One of the first tasks facing the committee was defining the terms related to its charge. The phrase "community-based, non-clinical prevention policy and wellness strategies" appears in the Statement of Task. This phrase has been shortened for purposes of this report to *community-based prevention*. The committee concluded that community-based prevention interventions are population-based interventions that are aimed at preventing the onset of disease, stopping or slowing the progress of disease, reducing or eliminating the negative consequences of disease, increasing healthful behaviors that result in improvements in health and well-being, or decreasing disparities that result in an inequitable distribution of health. The committee also concluded that, in addition to a focus on population health, community-based prevention interventions also may address changes in the social and physical environment, involve intersectoral action, highlight community participation and empowerment, emphasize context, or include a systems approach.

The committee uses the term *community* to mean any group of people who share geographic space, interests, goals, or history. A further discussion of community can be found in Chapter 2.

The *value* of an intervention, for purposes of this report, is defined as its benefits minus its harms and costs. There are expanded discussions of the concept of value at the end of Chapter 1 and in Chapter 4.

The committee concluded that a *framework for assessing value* is a structure for gathering and processing information to aid intelligent decision making and, more specifically, to help decide whether an activity or intervention is worthwhile. A framework for assessing value can aid decision making by

- requiring that goals be stated clearly;
- integrating incomplete and sometimes conflicting information and beliefs;
- avoiding decision making based on arbitrary impressions or self-interest;
- clarifying trade-offs;
- promoting transparency; and
- identifying and helping to work through legitimate sources of disagreement.

DOMAINS OF VALUE

The committee was asked to develop a framework for assessing the value of community-based prevention. Clearly, a major outcome of community-based prevention is its impact on health. However, because of the way in which community-based prevention is designed and developed (e.g., often to address the social and environmental determinants of health), the impacts of these interventions can go beyond health effects. Therefore, a framework for valuing community-based prevention needs to take into account not only the outcomes in the domain of health, but also outcomes in areas other than health. A framework that does not take into account and value non-health outcomes would be counting all the costs but not all the benefits, thereby providing an inaccurate and inadequate picture of the value of community-based prevention. Decision makers, funders, and stakeholders will all benefit from an approach that looks not just at health impacts, but at other impacts as well, and thus assesses the true value of community-based prevention.

The committee concluded that the outcomes of community-based prevention interventions can be divided into three distinct but interrelated categories, or *domains of value*: health, community well-being, and community process. The committee is aware that health is a component of well-being but for the purposes of this report the health component is separated from other elements of community well-being because health is a particular outcome of interest. By valuing these domains one can account for all of the potential harms and benefits of community-based prevention interventions as well as the possible savings and costs associated with the interventions. Chapter 3 provides an in-depth exploration of each of these domains of value; a brief summary is provided below. Many elements in each of the domains can be valued, and the ones selected will depend on the intervention of interest and on its implementation. The committee has identified one element—equity—that crosses all three domains.

The domain of *health* (both physical and mental) includes changes in the incidence and prevalence of disease, declines in mortality, and increases in health-related quality of life. More specifically, measures of physical health include mortality, morbidity, and functional capability. Measures of mental health include cognition, individual resilience or emotional reserves, mortality from such causes as suicide, morbidity (e.g., depression), and socio-emotional health-related quality of life (e.g., stress, behaviors, injuries, and perceptions of health).

Community well-being includes social norms, how people relate to each other and to their surroundings, and how much investment they are willing to make in themselves and in the people around them. Elements of community well-being include wealth and income, education, employment, crime, transportation, housing, worksites, food, social support and social networks, and health care, among others. These elements are produced, reproduced, and transformed by the practice of individuals in the community. Community well-being includes the physical as well as the social and economic environments that affect the health of individuals and populations, directly and indirectly.

The domain of *community process* includes local leadership development, skill building, civic engagement or participation, community representation, and community history, among others. Community processes typically have a sequence of activities that incorporate learning about various options available for health improvement, deliberations associated with the selection of one or more options, consideration of the appropriate methods to implement the health improvement initiatives, and critical reflection on the entire process. Not only can the way that decisions are made and carried out be important to the success of a program or policy—and thus to community well-being—it can also have a direct impact on well-being through benefits of broad participation and buy-in to decisions.

FRAMEWORK FOR VALUING

The committee concluded that a framework for valuing community-based prevention programs and policies should meet at least three criteria. First, the framework should account for benefits and harms in the three domains of health, community well-being, and community process. Community-based prevention can create value not only through improvements in the health of individuals but also by increasing the investment that individuals are willing and able to make in themselves, in their family and neighbors, and in their environment. Furthermore, community-based prevention involves decisions among groups of people about how to live in society, how the physical environment is built, what food is served in schools, and so on. Thus, the process by which interventions are decided upon and undertaken needs to be treated as a valued outcome. If a community decides to tell people what they can or cannot do, or what they should or should not do, the decisions need to have the legitimacy—the added value—that comes from an open and inclusive group decision-making process.

Second, the framework should consider the resources used and compare benefits and harms with those resources. To make that comparison and to compare different interventions with each other, it is essential to know not just that some benefit is likely but also the magnitude of the benefits and of the associated costs for each intervention.

Finally, the framework needs to be sensitive to differences among communities and to take them into account in valuing community-based prevention. In part, this reflects the reality that, because communities vary so much in their characteristics, the causal links between interventions and valued outcomes may be different for different communities.

None of the frameworks analyzed by the committee meets the criteria described above. (For a detailed discussion of the analysis, see Chapter 4.) Therefore, the committee concluded that a new framework was needed to assess the value of community-based prevention interventions.

The goals of the framework (Figure S-1) proposed by the committee are (1) to incorporate the full scope of benefits into the value of interventions,

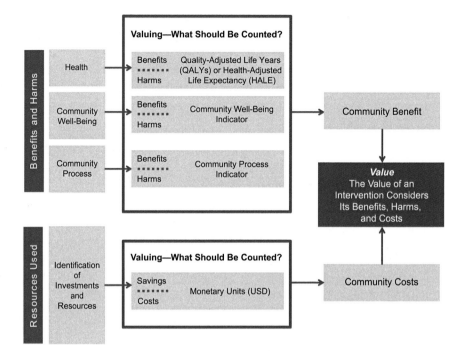

FIGURE S-1 Conceptual framework for valuing community-based prevention interventions.

so that in addition to health benefits and harms, the benefits and harms from community well-being and community process are included; (2) to emphasize that value requires a comparison of the benefits and harms of an intervention in relation to the resources used for the intervention; (3) to allow the specific characteristics and context of individual communities to be reflected in the valuation of community-based prevention; (4) to promote the quantification of value in terms of projected or actual changes due to the intervention; and (5) to encourage the development of evidence in order to make understanding the effects of interventions easier and more reliable. The valuation of community-based prevention interventions should be done with a comprehensive perspective; that is, the measurement of benefits, harms, and resources should include impacts on all members of the community as well as on stakeholders who may be outside the community. As illustrated in the framework, the measurement of benefits and harms should occur in the domains of health, community well-being, and community process. Resources used are a fourth major category to be considered in valuing community-based prevention. A further discussion of costs appears in Chapter 3 and in Box 5-1.

Recommendation 1: The committee recommends that those seeking to assign value to community-based prevention interventions take a comprehensive view that includes the benefits and harms in the three major domains of health, community well-being, and community process as well as the resource use associated with such interventions.

There are a variety of sources of data on health, including surveys (e.g., the National Health Interview Survey and the Behavioral Risk Factor Surveillance System), cohort studies (e.g., the Framingham Heart Study), registries, health services data, and vital statistics. Unfortunately, there are several limitations when attempting to use these data for local, community-based measurement. Identifying measures and sources of information for community well-being and community process elements is even more challenging than identifying these items for health. Such efforts will require an increased focus on identifying appropriate information gaps and data sources.

Recommendation 2: The committee recommends that the CDC
a. develop an inventory of existing data sources for health, community well-being, and community process;
b. identify gaps in data sources; and
c. develop data sources to fill those gaps.

Choosing among community-based prevention policies and programs can be difficult when programs have so many effects and those effects take so many different forms (see Chapter 3 for further discussion). The larger the menu of interventions and the larger the number of valued outcomes, the more difficult the choices become.

The committee proposes four indicators to assess the value of community-based prevention: changes in health, changes in community well-being, changes in community process, and changes in resources used. Health outcomes in the population can be valued with the well developed and widely used quality-adjusted life years (QALYs) or health-adjusted life expectancy (HALE). However, metrics for valuing community well-being and community process are yet to be developed. The committee is aware that the Centers for Disease Control and Prevention (CDC) has initiated efforts in these areas. Measures of community well-being (e.g., the Urban Hardship Index, Community Well-Being Indices, and county health rankings) have been developed and could serve as a starting point, but they have significant limitations in scope.

The committee views the development of a single indicator of community benefit comparable to QALYs or HALE for health as a long-term goal. The committee recognizes that developing this single indicator is a complex task that will require expertise from many different fields. The National Prevention, Health Promotion, and Public Health Council (Prevention Council), an interagency group established by the Patient Protection and Affordable Care Act and chaired by the Surgeon General, recognizes that the health of a community is influenced by a number of factors outside of the health care and public health sectors, including education, housing, and transportation. Such a group is well positioned to encourage the research needed by the many different sectors that need to be involved in developing a community benefit indicator.

> **Recommendation 3: The committee recommends that the National Prevention, Health Promotion, and Public Health Council and other public and private sponsors support research aimed at developing**
> a.   **a single metric for appraising a community's well-being,**
> b.   **a single metric for appraising community processes, and**
> c.   **a single metric for combining indicators of community well-being and community process with health into a single indicator of community benefit that can be considered in the context of costs and used to determine the value of a community-based prevention intervention.**

Given that the outcomes in the four domains are—or will be, once they are developed—measured in different units, a single indicator of the value of community-based prevention is currently not possible. However, in the framework depicted in Figure S-1, if the indicator of *community benefit* is considered alongside the *community cost* indicator (which is suggested to be expressed in dollars or other currency), then value may be expressed as units of *community benefit per dollar*. The proposed indicators are a first step toward a possible future overall summary measure.

The value of a community-based prevention intervention reflects its impact in relation to what would have happened in its absence or in relation to an alternative community-based prevention intervention. It is therefore important to assess the actual changes that are projected to occur as a result of an intervention.

> **Recommendation 4: The committee recommends that those assessing value should include in their assessments the expected or demonstrated changes, both positive and negative, that result from the intervention.**

Understanding what the community cares about is critical for designing and proposing interventions that address areas of importance to the community. Such an assessment will not only identify important health (and non-health) factors in the community but also those factors where improvement is preferred by community members. What is important for one community may not be important for another.

> **Recommendation 5: The committee recommends that those involved in decision making ensure that the elements included in valuing community-based prevention interventions reflect the preferences of an inclusive range of stakeholders.**

One dimension of the health outcomes that affects value is the possible conflict between equity and improving aggregate health for a population. Sometimes these two goals of health policy pull in the same direction, and sometimes they conflict. A community-based prevention intervention may be good at improving aggregate health, but it may have a bigger effect on those already better off in some important way, e.g., by income, residential location, or occupational status, and this may increase health disparities. The degree to which people are willing to trade off increased inequality for aggregate improvement may vary significantly. Reasonable disagreement about how to weigh these two values may persist, and the framework can make the source of that disagreement more visible.

The persistence of such disagreement around values suggests there may be a legitimacy problem for decision makers; even if they are the appropriate authorities for making such decisions, they must make them in the "right" way if legitimacy is to be obtained. Their process should search for rationales that take the relevant values into consideration, and the rationales must explain the basis for giving them the weight that the decision reflects. The framework emphasizes the importance of transparency, and one reason is that transparency improves the deliberative process. A transparent search for the value of an intervention is one key aspect of a process that arguably enhances legitimacy.

> **Recommendation 6: The committee recommends that, to assure transparency,**
> a. **analysts make publicly available the evidence used for valuation and provide estimates of the uncertainty of their results, and**
> b. **decision makers make publicly available the rationale for their decisions.**

IMPLICATIONS FOR POLICY

As with the frameworks discussed in Chapter 4, the committee's framework has limitations. The framework presented in this report is in its very early stages, and so its near-term impact on policy making is likely to be limited. Because of the importance of contextual factors and the limited scope and generalizability of evidence on the effects of community-based prevention, the framework does not yet provide a detailed roadmap for valuation. The comprehensive data necessary to measure tangible benefits adequately are often not available, and the measurement of the many intangible benefits is not yet well developed. Such a broadly inclusive framework may seem overly abstract or unreliable to some observers. As the framework is applied, new measures and data sources will need to be developed, as will an appropriate methodology for creating valid single indicators for community well-being and community process. Old measures and data sources will need to be applied in new ways, a process that will take time to establish validity and gain acceptance. The committee has recommended several steps that can be taken to promote progress on these fronts. Although much work remains, the committee's proposed framework is designed to capture the value of community-based prevention by taking a comprehensive approach, comparing benefits, harms, and resources used in three domains, and taking into account community context.

Additional efforts will be required to build consensus that the outcomes on which the framework focuses (health, community well-being, community process, and resources used) are broadly important, and not just the narrow interest of a specific group. It will also be important to validate the framework by showing repeatedly that it correctly distinguishes between interventions that improve community well-being and those that do not. This process of validation will almost certainly entail refinement of the framework as well as an expansion of the underlying base of evidence.

Formal incorporation of the framework into the policy-making process could consist of a requirement that legislative or grant proposals be accompanied by an objective impact assessment based on the framework or a requirement that executive-branch agencies use the framework in evaluating the output of their programs. Another way to give the framework a formal role would be to require that discretionary funding be distributed according to valuations that use the framework. Although that type of role may be many years off, the existing frameworks described in Chapter 4 provide clear precedents for such a progression.

The chapters of the report expand on the issues and findings discussed in this summary. Chapter 1 reviews the committee charge and definitions, explores why community-based prevention is important, examines how community-based prevention differs from clinical prevention efforts, and discusses issues associated with attempting to assign value. Chapter 2 expands on the discussion of community, provides a brief historical perspective of community interventions, discusses four approaches to community-based prevention, reviews models for implementation that represent the current state of the field, identifies important features of community-based prevention, and examines issues associated with evaluating the effectiveness of such programs. In Chapter 3, the committee examines how methods from systems science can be applied to community-based prevention, discusses how such methods can be used to clarify and quantify the relationships among variables, identifies domains of value for community-based prevention, and discusses costs to consider in valuing. Chapter 4 provides a list of elements that a framework for assessing value should possess, examines how a framework for valuing resides within a decision-making context, reviews eight frameworks currently used to assess community-based prevention, and discusses the strengths and limitations of each for addressing the special characteristics of community-based prevention. In Chapter 5, the committee lays out its vision for the future of valuing community-based prevention.

1

Introduction

This chapter begins by describing the scope of work for the study, then defines the terms the committee used to conduct its work, and, finally, discusses why community-based prevention is important and how it differs from other health improvement efforts. Some individuals believe the existing frameworks for valuing community-based prevention are flawed and prone to understating its benefits; others disagree or are uncertain. Committee members brought very different perspectives and areas of expertise to the discussion, with backgrounds that included public health, community health promotion, ethics, economics, workplace wellness, and government budget analysis. This report attempts the difficult task of blending those perspectives.

COMMITTEE CHARGE

Four foundations—the California Endowment, the de Beaumont Foundation, the Robert Wood Johnson Foundation, and the W.K. Kellogg Foundation—asked the Institute of Medicine to convene an expert committee to develop a framework for assessing the value of community-based, non-clinical prevention policies and wellness strategies, especially those targeting the prevention of long-term, chronic diseases. The committee's task was as follows:

- Define "community-based, non-clinical prevention policy and wellness strategies";

- Define "value" for community-based, non-clinical prevention policy and wellness strategies;
- Analyze current frameworks used to assess the value of community-based, non-clinical prevention policies and wellness strategies, including
  - o the methodologies and measures used and
  - o the short- and long-term impacts of such prevention policy and wellness strategies on communities, including health care spending and public health; and
- If warranted, propose a new framework or frameworks that capture the breadth and complexity of community-based, non-clinical prevention policies and wellness strategies, including interventions that target specific behaviors and health outcomes.

The framework should

- consider the sources of data that are needed and available;
- consider the concepts of generalization, scaling up, and sustainability of programs; and
- address national and state policy implications associated with implementing the framework.

The committee assembled to respond to the charge from the sponsors was composed of experts spanning different disciplines ranging from economics and program evaluation to community-based providers. Over the course of this 20-month study the committee met six times in person, participated in many conference calls, and held three information-gathering workshops. During the workshops, committee members heard from members of the prevention community as well as experts in the field of valuing different types of interventions, including interventions in the fields of education and housing.

DEFINITIONS

The committee's charge directs it to define "community-based, non-clinical prevention policy and wellness strategies" and also to define "value" for these policies and strategies. Through the course of its work the committee also used several other terms that may require clarification; in such cases definitions have been given in both the text of the report and in the glossary in Appendix A.

The phrase "community-based, non-clinical prevention policy and wellness strategies" appears in the Statement of Task. This phrase has been shortened for the purposes of this report to *community-based prevention*.

Community-based prevention includes programs and policies that are aimed at

- preventing the onset of disease,
- stopping or slowing the progress of disease,
- reducing or eliminating the negative consequences of disease,
- increasing healthful behaviors that result in improvements in health and well-being, or
- decreasing disparities that result in an inequitable distribution of health.

Community-based prevention is not primarily based on clinical services, although it may involve services provided by health professionals in clinical settings. The charge to the committee requested that special attention be given to the prevention of long-term, chronic diseases. Such a focus does not negate the fact that other community-based prevention efforts, such as those directed at unintended and intended injuries and mental health, are also important areas for attention.

The *value* of an intervention, for the purposes of this report, is defined as its benefits minus its harms and costs. There is an expanded discussion of the concept of value at the end of this chapter and in Chapter 4.

Community has been defined in a variety of ways. The committee uses the term community to mean any group of people who share geographic space, interests, goals, or history. It includes the built environment, social networks, and the organizations and institutions that sustain the individual and collective life of the community. Chapter 2 contains an expanded discussion of the concept of community.

A community-based prevention *program* is a coordinated activity or set of activities, such as an educational campaign against smoking, improvements to the built environment to encourage physical activity, a chronic disease education and awareness campaign to improve self-management, or a combination of such interventions, that is intended to accomplish a health objective or outcome. A *policy* is a rule or set of guidelines, such as nutritional standards for school lunches. An *intervention* is an umbrella term used to mean either a program or a policy with the goal of improving health. A *strategy* is the method through which programs are implemented, such as television advertisements warning of the dangers of smoking, construction of a bike path, or conducting disease management workshops in churches.

WHY IS COMMUNITY-BASED PREVENTION IMPORTANT?

Early health-promotion efforts emphasized meeting basic human needs for clean water, adequate nutrition, and shelter. In 1900 a third of all deaths in the United States were due to pneumonia, tuberculosis (TB), diarrhea and enteritis, and diphtheria. Children suffered high rates of morbidity and mortality, with 40 percent of deaths from those four causes occurring among children under five (CDC, 1999), and children under five accounting for a third of all deaths from all causes.

Over the past century major strides were made in improving the health of the public through population-level efforts that were implemented in individual communities. The reduction in premature mortality from TB brought about by community-based prevention is a dramatic example. In 1900 mortality rates from TB were 194 per 100,000. By 1940, before antibiotics for TB were available, the rate had dropped to 46 deaths for every 100,000 people living in the United States. The decrease was due to community-level infection control measures instituted by local health departments combined with improvements in housing (including reducing the level of crowding) and better nutrition (CDC, 1999). Large-scale public health initiatives, such as public sewer projects, chlorination of public water supplies, and food safety requirements, greatly reduced the exposure of the public to infectious organisms and reduced the incidence of such diseases as cholera, typhus, and TB (Turnock, 2009).

In the mid-20th century a new approach to improving health was made possible by the development of effective antibiotics and a new generation of vaccines combined with the professionalization of medicine. Since then, society has invested substantially in clinical interventions and strategies to improve health. This investment includes everything from the training of physicians, nurses, and other health professionals to the financing of expansions of hospital capacity and the development of new drug thera-pies, medical devices, and surgical techniques. Researchers have developed and fine-tuned frameworks such as randomized controlled trials and cost-effectiveness analysis for assessing the value of these clinical activities.

Decent housing, clean air and water, effective sanitation, and food safety have become such a part of our culture and public infrastructure that they are no longer thought of as health endeavors. Yet, the initiatives that led to these conditions brought about dramatic improvements in health. As we begin the 21st century there is growing recognition that the next stage of improving health and preventing disease will involve a renewed emphasis on population-level, non-clinical strategies. The committee expects that in the coming decades health practitioners and scholars will propose, develop, and implement more programs and policies designed to improve health at the community level; thus, a framework to evaluate their success and to compare them to other interventions is needed.

HOW IS COMMUNITY-BASED PREVENTION DIFFERENT?

Community-based prevention requires cultural, social, and environmental changes, much like the extensive changes in water, sanitation and housing, and nutrition that occurred in the first half of the 20th century. As discussed earlier, improving health and preventing disease does not occur solely in the patient's examination room; it also takes place in the community of patients and their families, friends and neighbors, employers, teachers, and storekeepers. People's socioeconomic status, social context, and physical and cultural environment influence their health both directly and, through behavioral changes and lifestyle development and reinforcement, indirectly (Box 1-1) (Adler et al., 2008; Berkman and Glass, 2000; Berkman and Kawachi, 2000). In addition, these factors can moderate and mediate the effects of clinical interventions on health (IOM, 2006).

During the second half of the 20th century, much of the focus of chronic disease epidemiology and prevention research was on individual lifestyle and behaviors, with the notable exception of tobacco control. In recent decades, however, research has demonstrated that behavioral choices are shaped and modulated by the environments in which individuals live (Adler et al., 2008; Antonovsky, 1967; Berkman and Glass, 2000; Cohen et al., 2000; Eller et al., 2008; Kawachi and Berkman, 2001, 2003; Marmot and Wilkinson, 1999; Stansfeld et al., 1999). Thus, for example, efforts to prevent obesity-related conditions might have limited success if they do not take into consideration the social and built-environment characteristics that might act as incentives or barriers to the dietary and physical activity choices that individuals make, and, indeed, recent initiatives in obesity control have been doing exactly that (e.g., Mercer et al., 2003; Sallis et al., 2006; Storey et al., 2003). Likewise, suicide, the 10th-leading cause of death among Americans, is tied to mental illness, also a long-term chronic disease that is clearly influenced by environment and social determinants (Galea et al., 2005; Huey and McNulty, 2005; Woo et al., 2012).

Clinical preventive interventions such as screening for conditions prior to the appearance of symptoms are important preventive services. For example, colonoscopies and mammograms have succeeded in identifying the potential for disease and led to early treatment to prevent occurrence. Screening, however, identifies problems that exist after the disease or its precursors are present (e.g., polyps in the colon or lumps in the breast) and is directed at individuals. Primary prevention, which addresses risk factors before disease occurs, is increasingly recognized as important (Haddix et al., 2003). It is more desirable to prevent obesity than to treat diabetes, yet delivering community-based prevention interventions is often more difficult to fund and staff than providing clinical interventions.

BOX 1-1
Disparities in Health

Chronic disease and its precursors are not distributed evenly across the population but are more likely to be present in minority and lower socioeconomic status (SES) populations (IOM, 2009, 2011). For example, significant differences in life expectancy remain between blacks and whites (CDC, 2011). Racial and ethnic disparities in health have more to do with differences in physical and social contexts than with individual biology and behavior. Some researchers have concluded that individuals' zip codes have a greater impact on their health than their genetic codes (RWJF, 2008). For example, in 2001 Diez-Roux and colleagues found that the neighborhood of residence had an impact on the risk of coronary heart disease even after controlling for income, education, and occupation (Diez-Roux et al., 2001).

The social determinants that lead to poor health—poverty, lower levels of education, poor housing and nutrition, limited health literacy—are more likely to be present in populations marginalized by prejudice and poverty. The risk factors that arise from these determinants—obesity, tobacco and drug use, stress, depression, occupational and other environmental exposures—are also more prevalent, as are the diseases that result (RWJF, 2008).

Even when other risk factors have been accounted for, however, SES appears to have an effect on health. The Whitehall II Study of British civil servants by Michael Marmot and colleagues (1991) demonstrated that, despite universal access to health care, there was a stepwise gradient of health, with the higher-grade civil servants having better health and persons in the top ranks of Whitehall being the healthiest of all. The researchers discovered that about 20 percent of the variance in health status and life expectancy between grades could not be explained by the usual risk factors for poor health. This relationship between social status and health is referred to as *the social gradient in health.* Further analysis of the data on the effect of biological and behavioral factors on the risk of coronary heart disease within the Whitehall cohort showed that only about 60 percent of the social gradient could be explained by these factors (Marmot, 2004). Potential social explanations for these differences include the concepts of self-efficacy and empowerment, but uncertainty remains about the biological pathways that might underlie the influence of such social factors on health.

WHY IS IT SO HARD TO ASSESS THE VALUE OF COMMUNITY-BASED PREVENTION?

Policies and programs to avoid further deterioration of health or death once a person is ill are generally seen as reasonable. However, preventing illness requires that society invest the financial and other resources necessary to make the required changes in individual and community life *before* someone becomes sick, and this means that some of the persons who receive the intervention—and share the costs for it—would never have become sick anyway. Thus it can be easier to make the case for improving an individual's health, where the cost–benefit relationship is clearer, than it is to make the case for community-based prevention, especially to individuals who perceive their own risk of illness as low.

In contrast to individuals who need treatment because they are ill, those who avoid an illness due to a prevention program are not individually identifiable and thus may not realize that they have benefited. The costs of these programs are immediate, but the benefits are often deferred to the future. Furthermore, members of the community can vary in their priorities and principles. Disagreements over the merits of a program or policy objectives and disputes about the methods used to implement a program also hinder funding of some community activities.

The Concept of Value

Assessing the value of something requires first defining value conceptually and then measuring it. On both counts, community-based prevention is complex (see Box 1-2). The committee identified several conceptual issues that make defining value difficult.

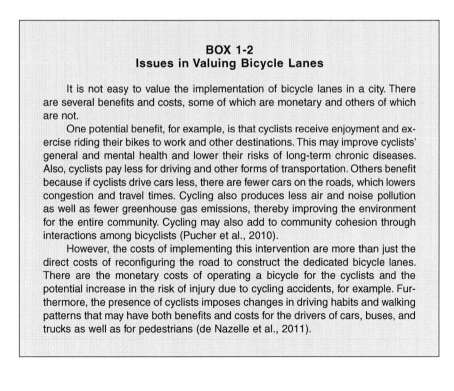

BOX 1-2
Issues in Valuing Bicycle Lanes

It is not easy to value the implementation of bicycle lanes in a city. There are several benefits and costs, some of which are monetary and others of which are not.

One potential benefit, for example, is that cyclists receive enjoyment and exercise riding their bikes to work and other destinations. This may improve cyclists' general and mental health and lower their risks of long-term chronic diseases. Also, cyclists pay less for driving and other forms of transportation. Others benefit because if cyclists drive cars less, there are fewer cars on the roads, which lowers congestion and travel times. Cycling also produces less air and noise pollution as well as fewer greenhouse gas emissions, thereby improving the environment for the entire community. Cycling may also add to community cohesion through interactions among bicyclists (Pucher et al., 2010).

However, the costs of implementing this intervention are more than just the direct costs of reconfiguring the road to construct the dedicated bicycle lanes. There are the monetary costs of operating a bicycle for the cyclists and the potential increase in the risk of injury due to cycling accidents, for example. Furthermore, the presence of cyclists imposes changes in driving habits and walking patterns that may have both benefits and costs for the drivers of cars, buses, and trucks as well as for pedestrians (de Nazelle et al., 2011).

Whose values? The value of an intervention depends on one's perspective and on one's beliefs and priorities. A program may have a very different value depending on whether the perspective is that of the federal budget, of a specific employer, of specific segments of society or a particular community, or of society in general. For example, the success of tobacco control is partly due to smoking restrictions in such places as workplaces, restaurants, and airplanes. To a nonsmoker with a generally positive view of regulation, such restrictions are valuable. To others, such as business owners who fear losing customers, such restrictions can be seen as harmful.

Values diverge on other dimensions as well. Consider needle exchange programs. Public health workers may support such programs because research has shown that they reduce the transmission of HIV (NIH, 1997). But others in the community may object because they view these programs as facilitating illegal drug use. Both groups want to discourage these activities but evaluate the trade-offs between the benefits and harms differently. To be successful, complex programs require the collaboration or at least cooperation of many sectors and organizations that may have differing values.

To monetize, or not to monetize. One approach to assessing the value of something is to measure, in dollar terms, its impacts in terms of benefits and costs. Some things are naturally monetized, such as the time spent by a paid community health educator. Other things are much more difficult, but not necessarily impossible, to monetize, such as the value of increased social cohesion. To some, the monetized approach allows a straightforward assessment of whether an intervention is worth undertaking. Monetization strikes others as misguided or wrong.

To summarize, or not to summarize. Policy makers crave simple summaries of a proposal's impact—for example, how many lives will be saved and how many dollars the intervention will cost. Community-based prevention efforts are difficult to summarize since their effects can span financial, social, environmental, business, and ethical domains. The value of an intervention also depends critically on where and how well it is carried out.

A ROADMAP FOR THE REST OF THE REPORT

In this chapter, the committee has discussed the committee charge, defined important terms, examined why community-based prevention is important and how it differs from other prevention approaches, and explored the concept and issues involved in valuing such programs and policies. Chapter 2 expands on the discussion of community, provides a brief historical perspective of community interventions, discusses four approaches to community-based prevention, reviews the models for implementation that represent the current state of the field, identifies key features of community-based prevention, and examines issues associated with evaluating the effectiveness of such programs.

In Chapter 3 the committee examines how methods from systems science can be applied to community-based prevention, discusses how such methods can be used to clarify and quantify the relationships among variables, and identifies outcomes or domains of value for community-based prevention. Chapter 4 provides a list of elements that a framework for assessing value should possess, examines how a framework for valuing resides within a decision-making context, reviews eight frameworks currently used to assess community-based prevention, and discusses the strengths and limitations of each for addressing the special characteristics of community-based prevention. In Chapter 5 the committee lays out its vision for the future of valuing community-based prevention.

REFERENCES

Adler, N., A. Singh-Manoux, J. Schwartz, J. Stewart, K. Matthews, and M. G. Marmot. 2008. Social status and health: A comparison of British civil servants in Whitehall II with European- and African-Americans in CARDIA. *Social Science and Medicine* 66(5):1034-1045.

Antonovsky, A. 1967. Social class, life expectancy and overall mortality. *Milbank Memorial Fund Quarterly* 45(2):31-73.

Berkman, L., and T. A. Glass. 2000. Social integration, social networks, social support, and health. In *Social epidemiology*, edited by L. Berkman and I. Kawachi. New York: Oxford University Press. Pp. 137-173.

Berkman, L., and I. Kawachi (Eds.). 2000. *Social epidemiology*. New York: Oxford University Press.

CDC (Centers for Disease Control and Prevention). 1999. Ten great public health achievements—United States, 1900-1999. *Morbidity and Mortality Weekly Report* 48(12):241.

CDC. 2011. Deaths: Preliminary data for 2009. *National Vital Statistics Reports* 59(4).

Cohen, S., I. Brissette, D. P. Skoner, and W. J. Doyle. 2000. Social integration and health: The case of the common cold. *Journal of Social Structure* 1(3):1-7.

de Nazelle, A., M. J. Nieuwenhuijsen, J. M. Antó, M. Brauer, D. Briggs, C. Braun-Fahrlander, N. Cavill, A. R. Cooper, H. Desqueyroux, S. Fruin, G. Hoek, L. I. Panis, N. Janssen, M. Jerrett, M. Joffe, Z. J. Andersen, E. van Kempen, S. Kingham, N. Kubesch, K. M. Leyden, J. D. Marshall, J. Matamala, G. Mellios, M. Mendez, H. Nassif, D. Ogilvie, R. Peiró, K. Pérez, A. Rabl, M. Ragettli, D. Rodríguez, D. Rojas, P. Ruiz, J. F. Sallis, J. Terwoert, J.-F. Toussaint, J. Tuomisto, M. Zuurbier, and E. Lebret. 2011. Improving health through policies that promote active travel: A review of evidence to support integrated health impact assessment. *Environment International* 37(4):766-777.

Diez-Roux, A. V, S. S. Merkin, D. Arnett, L. Chambless, M. Massing, F. J. Nieto, P. Sorlie, M. Szklo, H. A. Tyroler, and R. L. Watson. 2001. Neighborhood of residence and incidence of coronary heart disease. *New England Journal of Medicine* 345(2):99-106.

Eller, M., R. Holle, R. Landgraf, and A. Mielck. 2008. Social network effect on self-rated health in type 2 diabetic patients—results from a longitudinal population-based study. *International Journal of Public Health* 53(4):188-194.

Galea, S., J. Ahern, S. Rudenstine, Z. Wallace, and D. Vlahov. 2005. Urban built environment and depression: A multilevel analysis. *Journal of Epidemiology and Community Health* 59(10):822-827.

Haddix, A. C., S. M. Teutsch, and P. S. Corso. 2003. *Prevention effectiveness: A guide to decision analysis and economic evaluation.* New York: Oxford University Press.

Huey, M. P., and T. L. McNulty. 2005. Institutional conditions and prison suicide: Conditional effects of deprivation and overcrowding. *Prison Journal* 85(4):490-514.

IOM (Institute of Medicine). 2006. *Genes, behavior, and the social environment: Moving beyond the nature/nurture debate.* Washington, DC: The National Academies Press.

IOM. 2009. *State of the USA health indicators: Letter report.* Washington, DC: The National Academies Press.

IOM. 2011. *A nationwide framework for surveillance of cardiovascular and chronic lung diseases.* Washington, DC: The National Academies Press.

Kawachi, I., and L. Berkman. 2001. Social ties and mental health. *Journal of Urban Health* 78(3):458-467.

Kawachi, I., and L. Berkman. 2003. *Neighborhoods and health.* New York: Oxford University Press.

Marmot, M. 2004. *Status syndrome: How social standing affects our health and longevity.* New York: Times Books.

Marmot, M. G., and R. G. Wilkinson. 1999. *Social determinants of health.* Oxford: Oxford University Press.

Marmot, M. G., G. D. Smith, S. Stansfeld, C. Patel, F. North, J. Head, I. White, E. Brunner, and A. Feeney. 1991. Health inequalities among British civil servants: The Whitehall II study. *Lancet* 337(8754):1387-1393.

Mercer, S. L., L. W. Green, A. C. Rosenthal, C. G. Husten, L. K. Khan, and W. H. Dietz. 2003. Possible lessons from the tobacco experience for obesity control. *American Journal of Clinical Nutrition* 77(4):1073S-1082S.

NIH (National Institutes of Health). 1997. *Consensus Development Statement on Interventions to Prevent HIV Risk Behaviors.* http://consensus.nih.gov/1997/1997PreventHIVRisk104html.htm (accessed July 6, 2012).

Pucher, J., R. Buehler, D. R. Bassett, and A. L. Dannenberg. 2010. Walking and cycling to health: A comparative analysis of city, state, and international data. *American Journal of Public Health* 100(10):1986-1992.

RWJF (Robert Wood Johnson Foundation). 2008. *Overcoming Obstacles to Health: Report from the Robert Wood Johnson Foundation to the Commission to Build a Healthier America.* Princeton, NJ: RWJF.

Sallis, J. F., R. B. Cervero, W. Ascher, K. A. Henderson, M. K. Kraft, and J. Kerr. 2006. An ecological approach to creating active living communities. *Annual Review of Public Health* 27:297-322.

Stansfeld, S., J. Head, and J. Ferrie. 1999. Short-term disability, sickness absence, and social gradients in the Whitehall II study. *International Journal of Law and Psychiatry* 22(5-6):425-439.

Storey, M. L., R. A. Forshee, A. R. Waever, and W. R. Sansalone. 2003. Demographic and lifestyle factors associated with body mass index among children and adolescents. *International Journal of Food Sciences and Nutrition* 54(6):491.

Turnock, B. H. 2009. *Public Health: What It Is and How It Works,* 4th ed. Sudbury, MA: Jones and Bartlett Publishers.

Woo, J. M., O. Okusaga, and T. T. Postolache. 2012. Seasonality of suicidal behavior. *International Journal of Environmental Research and Public Health* 9(2):531-547.

2

Community-Based Prevention

For purposes of brevity and consistency, the committee has chosen to use the term "community-based prevention" to describe community-based prevention policies and wellness strategies. This chapter begins with a discussion of the terms "community," "community-based," and "community-placed." It then identifies important features of community-based prevention, gives a brief history of the development of community-based prevention programs, and describes strategies and a sampling of models used. The chapter also examines the evidence used and the difficulties inherent in the evaluation of effectiveness as well in describing results from some program evaluations.

COMMUNITY

Community means different things to different people in different contexts. For example, Cheadle and colleagues (1997) refer to community as a location or place. Brennan (2002) writes that "community may be a more abstract concept, such as a neighborhood, defined by a sense of identity or shared history with boundaries that are more fluid and not necessarily identified exactly the same by all members." For some, community may be defined by common beliefs or ideologies (e.g., religion or politics), by activity (e.g., swing dancing or running), by social responsibility, by race or ethnicity, by socioeconomic status, or by a sense of belonging (Israel et al., 1994; Patrick and Wickizer, 1995; Rossi, 2001).

For purposes of this report, community is defined as any group of people who share geographic space, interests, goals, or history. A community offers a diversity of potential targets for prevention and is often conceived of as an encompassing, proximal, and comprehensive structure that provides opportunities and resources that shape people's lifestyle (McIntyre and Ellaway, 2000). A community also offers the potential for pooling resources and for collaboration among community-based organizations, some of which are affiliates of state and national organizations that can channel resources to them in support of local initiatives and the evaluation of their innovations (Kreuter et al., 2000).

A distinction can be made between community-based prevention and community-placed prevention, or community interventions versus interventions in communities (Green and Kreuter, 2005), although both take a population-based approach. Community-based activity involves members of the affected community in the planning, development, implementation, and evaluation of programs and strategies (Cargo and Mercer, 2008). An example of this type of prevention effort is community-based participatory research, in which academic researchers—who are usually in control of the decisions on the research question, design, methods, and interpretation of results—invite or concede at least an equal partner role to community members in formulating, conducting, and interpreting the research. It is important to note that rarely are all members of a community involved and that for those who are, the level of involvement can vary tremendously.

Community-placed activities, on the other hand, are developed without the participation of members of the affected community at important stages of the project. While the program may be centrally planned, effort is expended to generate community support. An example of the community-placed approach is the YMCA diabetes prevention program that is being implemented in partnership with YMCAs across the country, some with more tailoring to the localities than others (Ritchie et al., 2010).

Although there are distinct differences between these two approaches to prevention, for purposes of this report key domains for valuing (discussed in Chapter 3) are common to both approaches. Therefore, the term "community-based prevention" is used to encompass both community-placed and community-based prevention programs, policies, and strategies.

IMPORTANT FEATURES OF
COMMUNITY-BASED PREVENTION

Over the past 50 years public health practice and research have contributed to developing and analyzing the characteristics that distinguish community-based prevention from other forms of action. Community-based prevention interventions focus on population health and, in addition, may address changes in the social and physical environment, involve intersectoral action, highlight community participation and empowerment, emphasize context, or include a systems approach.

Community-based prevention is not focused on changing individual characteristics. Rather, the focus is on *population health*, that is, on "the health outcomes of a group of individuals, including the distribution of such outcomes within the group" (Kindig and Stoddart, 2003). For example, implementing nutritional standards for a population is a community-based prevention intervention. Such standards require decision making by a school district and their development may include elected officials, parents, administrators, and students. They affect all of the students and parents in the school district. An individual buying a Stairmaster and using it at home is also taking part in a nonclinical prevention program, but it is not community-based. The owner of the Stairmaster need not consult the neighbors before purchasing it, nor are the neighbors helped by the purchase.

Changes in social and physical features of the environment constitute valued outcomes for community-based prevention because the distributions of risk factors, health outcomes, and wellness indicators in a population are largely shaped by social and physical environments. Research has shown that social characteristics such as socioeconomic status, social cohesion, social capital, and friendship networks are associated with health and well-being (Adler et al., 2008; Berkman and Kawachi, 2000). The same is true for such features of the natural and built physical environment as poor housing, increased levels of pollution, the presence of green spaces, quality of housing, the safety and pleasantness of the walking infrastructure, and many others (Gauderman et al., 2004; Handy, 2004; IOM, 2000a; Kawachi and Berkman, 2003; Nelson et al., 2006).

Research also has demonstrated that intersectoral action is an important component of interventions aimed at population health (Gibson et al., 2007; Kreisel and Schirnding, 1998). *Intersectoral action* refers to engaging and coordinating actors from a variety of relevant sectors in the planning, implementation, and governance of interventions. Because most of the social and environmental determinants of population health exist outside the sphere of influence of the health sector, such intersectoral partnerships are key processes by which changes in the main determinants of health can happen (Gibson et al., 2007).

The health in all policies (HiAP) approach to address the social determinants of health encourages governments to include multiple sectors (e.g., taxation, education, transportation) in programs and policies to improve population health (WHO, 2010). Examples can be found in the Institute of Medicine (IOM) report that examined the role of laws and other policies on the public's health. That report endorsed the potential of HiAP in population health improvement and provided examples of local, state, and federal-level collaboration among different sectors, including transportation, planning, and community development (IOM, 2011). The report also described a continuum of applications for HiAP, ranging from "do no harm" (i.e., consider the health effects of proposed policy in non-health areas) to a proactive approach to addressing the most distal determinants of health. Finally, the report recommended local planning processes modeled on the structure and role of the National Prevention, Health Promotion and Public Health Council, and designed to engage a variety of external stakeholders.

Community participation refers to the engagement of those affected in the process of transforming those conditions that influence community health. Participation can occur at various stages of the project and can also vary in intensity. It can involve the affected individuals themselves or spokespersons for them. In community interventions, participation often translates into volunteer work and other local resources that increase the potential intensity of the intervention.

Adapting community-based interventions to local conditions and context is an important feature of effective interventions and increases community ownership and buy in for the intervention (McLaren et al., 2007). However, it is insufficient to assume that community participation will result in change. Change is dependent on who participates and varies as leadership changes. Many times it is the "squeaky wheels" that persist and carry the day whether they are representative or not. These processes take a long time during which many things change, including broad secular changes like the local economy, leadership, availability of funding, etc. While engagement is indeed relevant to successful interventions, it is important to be aware that it is no panacea.

Empowerment refers to the ability of individuals or groups to exercise control over the conditions and circumstances that influence health and well-being. Intervention processes that promote empowerment and capacity development are also often participatory (Dressendorfer et al., 2005; Israel et al., 1994). It has been demonstrated that collective empowerment enables communities to better identify and solve their problems through more efficient processes of assessing needs and advocating for policies (Edmundo et al., 2005; Reininger et al., 2005).

The *context* within which community-based prevention is developed and implemented is also important. Intervention means there is an interruption of the normal evolution of events or trajectory, sometimes from outside the community. This outside trigger may be a funding opportunity or a policy or administrative initiative from another level of government or organization that resides outside the community of interest. Funding opportunities may come from various sources and be associated with other types of resources, such as access to technical expertise and knowledge. These triggers are external resources that can be invested in the solution of a problem or in the improvement of local conditions. Alternatively, the outside event might be a global or national trend, such as global warming or a pandemic that is threatening local communities.

Effective mechanisms for community-based prevention do not, however, reside solely in the external resources that constitute or support the intervention. Characteristics of the community in which the intervention will be implemented interact with those resources and include the cultural, social, political, and physical characteristics of the populations that are targeted by the intervention. These characteristics may also be transformed through the intervention process, increasingly blurring the distinction between the intervention (in the sense of the effective transformative mechanism), context, and intervention effect.

A *systems approach* is the final feature discussed here. (For more on the systems approach, see Chapter 3.) Comprehensive community-based prevention efforts provide for a combination of interventions that predispose, enable, and reinforce the behavioral and social changes that individuals and organizations need to make in order to successfully achieve health outcomes (Green and Kreuter, 2005; Wagner et al., 2000). They also encompass multiple sectors and multiple levels, as with state-level mass media and the local tailoring of interventions.

HISTORICAL PERSPECTIVE

Community-based prevention efforts aimed at addressing the living and working conditions that affect health are not new. As discussed in Chapter 1, the major causes of morbidity and mortality in the 19th century were communicable diseases. Early attempts to control these diseases focused on community-based prevention aimed at improving personal hygiene, housing and sanitary reforms, and laws to improve living conditions among poor urban dwellers. Other efforts focused on improving food and workplace safety. Population health in the United States improved dramatically because of these community-based efforts. As a result of these efforts as well as improvements in clinical prevention, chronic diseases and injuries have replaced communicable diseases as the leading causes of illness and mortality in the United States.

Just as the major causes of morbidity and mortality have changed, so too has our understanding of health and what makes people healthy or ill. In 1974 Marc Lalonde, Minister of National Health and Welfare Canada, presented a white paper that laid out the perspective that health is influenced by environment, lifestyle, human biology, and health care organization. Evans and Stoddart (1990) presented a more complex model of the determinants of health which included behavioral and biological responses to both the social and physical environments. The report *Gulf*

War Veterans: Measuring Health (IOM, 1999) proposed a framework for health that described how individual and environmental characteristics influence health-related quality of life. And a list of major health determinants assembled by Kaplan and colleagues (IOM, 2000b) included pathophysiological pathways, genetic and individual risk factors, social relationships, living conditions, neighborhoods and communities, institutions, and social and economic policies. In 2002, the IOM report *The Future of the Public's Health* developed a new model, adapted from Dahlgren and Whitehead (1991), that presented an ecological view of the determinants of health, discussed later in this chapter.

Research has documented the important effects that social determinants have on health, both directly and through their impact on other health determinants, such as risk factors (Berkman and Kawachi, 2000). It has long been known, for example, that people with greater socioeconomic status are healthier than those with lower status; that those with social support fare better, both physically and mentally, than those without; and that one's neighborhood and built environment affect one's health (Adler et al., 2008; Antonovsky, 1967; Berkman and Glass, 2000; Cohen et al., 2000; Eller et al., 2008; Kawachi and Berkman, 2001, 2003; Marmot and Wilkerson, 2000; Stansfeld et al., 1999). Such inequalities highlight the importance of focusing on social determinants when intervening to improve the health of individuals and communities.

In 1990, McGinnis and Foege (1993) estimated more than 50 percent of the deaths in the United States each year can be traced to tobacco use, alcohol consumption, a sedentary lifestyle, and a diet heavy in salt, sugar, and fat and low in fruits and vegetables. A later analysis by Mokdad and colleagues (2004, 2005) found that for the year 2000, 18.1 percent of U.S. deaths were attributable to tobacco, 15.2 percent to poor diet and physical inactivity, 3.5 percent to alcohol consumption, and other percentages, in decreasing order, were attributable to microbial agents, toxic agents, motor vehicle crashes, incidents involving firearms, sexual behaviors, and illicit use of drugs. Targeting interventions toward the conditions associated with today's challenges to living a healthy life requires an increased emphasis on the factors that affect these causes of morbidity and mortality, factors such as the social determinants of health.

Recent work in community-based prevention has also sought to address the distribution of health and risk factors in populations through programs, policies, and strategies that attempt to reduce social inequalities—or to mitigate their effect on health—and to strengthen the cultural assets of all groups (Bleich et al., 2011). Several approaches to health behavior change, discussed below, have contributed to the way in which current community-based prevention efforts are planned and implemented to address not only population-wide change, but also a reduction in the disparities among social groups.

Health Behavior Change

The U.S. Agricultural Extension Service produced a model of community diffusion and adoption of innovations that continues to inform and guide the planning of community health behavior programs (Brownson et al., 2012; Green et al., 2009; Lionberger, 1964; Rogers, 2002). At the level of individual behavior change, the diffusion model evolved to represent stages in the innovation-diffusion process. The translation of this model to community-based prevention has generally taken the form of interpreting each stage in the individual adoption model relative to the community supports it might need or the community efforts required to facilitate each phase (Rogers, 2002), as illustrated in Table 2-1.

A model for community-based prevention developed in the 1950s and 1960s grew out of efforts to increase both immunization coverage for mass poliomyelitis protection and mass screening for cancer and tuberculosis (Deasy, 1956; D'Onofrio, 1966; Hochbaum, 1956, 1959). This model, the Health Belief Model, was primarily a psychological model developed from community screening and immunization programs, but it became a part of community intervention models in that it provided a guide to planning the mass media component for recruitment of people for screening or immunization in community programs (Becker, 1974; Harrison et al., 1992; Janz and Becker, 1984).

Another development in the 1960s, which accompanied President Kennedy's New Frontier initiative and President Johnson's Great Society,

TABLE 2-1 Features of the Organization or Community Supporting States of the Individual Change Process

Phase in Psychological Process of Change	Supporting Features of Community
Exposure	Social setting with access to media
Attention	Interest of family, peers, and other significant persons
Comprehension	Group discussion and feedback, question and answer sessions
Belief	Direct persuasion and social influence, actions of informal leaders
Decision	Group decision making, public commitments, and repeated encouragement, which build self confidence
Learning	Demonstrated and guided practice with feedback and continued confidence, advice, and direct assistance

SOURCE: Green and McAlister, 1984.

War on Poverty, and civil rights initiatives, was the promotion of public participation in community health planning. Each legislative act of those initiatives carried the phrase "maximum feasible participation," which required 51 percent of the planning boards for local program entities to be nonprofessional residents of the community. Insufficient funding for these efforts, however, produced understaffed community agencies and programs. This led many of the agencies and programs to turn to their volunteer community planning participants to help staff the organizations. Daniel Patrick Moynihan (1969) referred to this as "maximum feasible misunderstanding" of the participatory principle. Citizen participation in planning community programs fell into some disrepute as a result, but the stage was set for a later revival of participatory principles in community health assessments, planning, research, and evaluation (Green, 1970b, 1986b).

In the 1970s and 1980s, as the growing experience with multisector community approaches took form with community health planning and regional medical programs, the principle of participation evolved from one emphasizing the generation of community support for centrally planned programs to a principle of involving the community in planning programs locally (Green, 1986a). As described by Hackett (1982), "It was from such principles that the modern strategy of community health in countries arose, which was adopted and put into practice by the World Health Organization and was presented at the Alma Ata Conference on Primary Health Care in 1978."

These moves away from individually focused clinical prevention strategies were not yet penetrating the chronic disease control field, however. In the 1970s the first trials aimed at reducing the prevalence of behavioral risk factors associated with cardiovascular disease (CVD) were based in clinical settings and were directed at patients who were at risk of developing CVD. For example, the Multiple Risk Factor Intervention Trial (MRFIT) randomly assigned about 13,000 men at high risk of coronary heart disease (CHD) either to usual care and medical follow-up or to a series of prevention interventions. However, the prevention interventions mainly consisted of the medical control of high blood pressure, smoking cessation sessions, and dietary counseling for lowering cholesterol level. Although the experimental group showed improvements in the prevalence of risk factors, notably reductions in smoking, such improvements were not significantly different from those observed in the control group. One hypothesis for this minimal difference was that community and mass media activities addressing these risk factors were taking hold, resulting in pervasive exposures of the control groups to influences as strong as the clinical interventions (Green and Richard, 1993).

While clinical approaches have important contributions to make in addressing risk factors, community-based prevention programs have three distinct strengths:

1. Community-based prevention is aimed at and implemented in a population. Therefore, all members of that population have access to the intervention. Clinical services, however, reach only those individuals who can afford and seek clinical services.
2. Because community strategies are directed at a population, they can reach individuals with varying levels of risk and, in particular, the large group of people who generally fall in the middle of a bell-shaped curve (Rose, 1992). Clinical services tend to be directed at changes for the relatively smaller number of high-risk individuals, those at the high end of the curve. This means they do not prevent individuals who are at lower risk from developing behaviors and lifestyles that will put them at higher risk (Syme, 1994).
3. Lifestyle and behavioral risk factors are shaped by environmental conditions that are not necessarily under the direct control of individuals or of their physicians (Cockerham et al., 1997; Frohlich et al., 2001; Kawachi and Berkman, 2003). Community-based prevention programs can be designed to affect environmental and social conditions that clinical services cannot.

The Settings Approach

As discussed above, clinical prevention alone is insufficient to modify behavioral risk factors at the level of populations. Complementary community-based prevention programs and policies can be implemented in workplaces, schools, families, and communities (Poland et al., 2000). Some settings (such as schools) provide a more or less captive pool of identifiable individuals who can be reached easily with an intervention as long as it does not require modifying environmental conditions (Richard et al., 1996). School immunization programs in which school registries and classrooms are used for the identification, gathering, and vaccination of children are an example of such prevention interventions in schools. By contrast, other interventions are designed to modify a setting's physical and social environmental conditions that influence the prevalence of risk factors. Prominent examples have been workplace bans on smoking, which protected workers from the secondhand smoke of other employees or of customers and also began to change norms about the acceptability of smoking in public places. Similarly, the banning of unhealthful products from vending machines in schools, and the construction of bike paths in urban areas has improved the health environments of children and adults.

APPROACHES TO COMMUNITY INTERVENTION

It is beyond the scope of this report to offer a full review of the approaches to community-based prevention aimed at altering the distribution of disease risk factors. However, this chapter does explore four categories of such efforts: the ecological approach, social marketing and public health education, health promotion, and policy change. Community-based prevention programs that combine these four approaches can produce systems changes that are comprehensive and that exhibit significant and durable effects on a population. For more discussion about systems, see Chapter 3.

Ecological

The first group of strategies is based on an ecological model of public health interventions. An ecological model (Figure 2-1) published in the report *Who Will Keep the Public Healthy?: Educating Public Health Professionals for the 21st Century* "assumes that health and well being are affected by the interaction among multiple determinants including biology, behavior, and the environment" (IOM, 2003, p. 32). A recognition of the multiple determinants of health, including the importance of the social and environmental determinants, is a key feature of the ecological approach. For community-based prevention interventions using the ecological approach, the interaction between levels of influence creates multiple opportunities for designing interventions to affect successive levels of the community structure (McLaren and Hawe, 2005). Various ecological models have been developed which incorporate concepts such as resources, social ecology, the life course and learning processes, and social context in order to demonstrate how the environment shapes individual behavior (Richard et al., 2011).

In addition to the development of interventions aimed at changing individual behaviors, the ecological approach can also be applied to affect collective behavior, organizational behavior, and the reciprocal relationship between the various levels via constraints and resources embedded in the structural features of the socio-cultural context (Stokols, 1992). Such a perspective integrates the approaches of individual behavioral interventions and interventions affecting the physical environment in an effort to focus action on the social environment to account for the needs of individuals and the resources available to address those needs (Stokols, 1996; Stokols et al., 1996). Several distinct uses of the ecological perspective have been described in the public health literature (IOM, 2003). They emphasize the need for interventions to target the various systems that influence behaviors (McLeroy et al., 1988; Richard et al., 1996; Stokols, 1996).

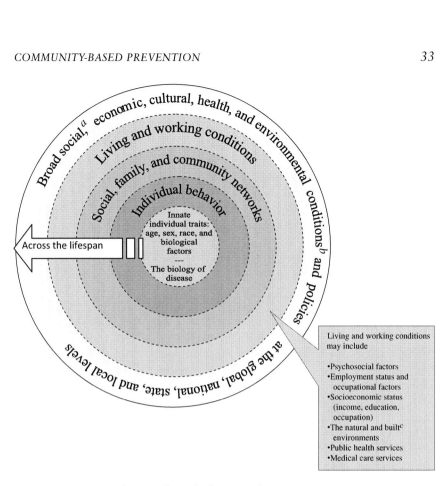

FIGURE 2-1 A guide to ecological planning of community prevention programs. NOTE: The dotted lines between levels of the model denote interaction effects between and among the various levels of health determinants (Worthman, 1999).

[a] Social conditions include, but are not limited to, economic inequality, urbanization, mobility, cultural values, attitudes, and policies related to discrimination and intolerance on the basis of race, gender, and other differences.

[b] Other conditions at the national level might include major sociopolitical shifts, such as recession, war, and governmental collapse.

[c] The built environment includes transportation, water and sanitation, housing, and other dimensions under the auspices of urban planning.

SOURCE: Adapted from Dahlgren and Whitehead, 1991.

Social Marketing and Public Health Education

Social marketing and education are strategies that seek to change people's knowledge and attitudes about health, risk factors, and determinants. At the most basic level, prevention interventions seek to increase people's awareness, knowledge, and attitudes about chronic disease risk factors and lifestyle based on the premise that knowing what is good for oneself is a necessary first step for behavior change. Such interventions work best when they focus in the short run on a single issue or behavior or else on a small set of interrelated disease-specific risk factors (e.g., Eriksen et al., 2007). (One notable exception is school health education, which has traditionally sought to build a cohesive body of personal health knowledge and competence.) Awareness and attitude-change programs in public health education have increasingly adopted the principles of social marketing, which is understood as a "process for influencing human behavior on a large scale, using marketing principles for the purpose of societal benefit" (Smith, 2000). The National Social Marketing Center in England defines social marketing as "the systematic application of marketing, along with other concepts and techniques, to achieve specific behavioral goals for a social good" (French, 2009; Reynolds, 2012).

A key feature of social marketing is the segmentation of the target group into individual homogenous audiences each with similar attitudes and beliefs (Diehr et al., 2011). Common bases for segmenting the target audience include attitudes, behaviors, demographics, epidemiology, geography, psychographics,[1] motives and benefits sought, and the stage of readiness for change (Donovan et al., 2010). In public health, social marketing has been conceptualized as a way to tackle the limitations of individual and small-group counseling and as a means to reach a broader segment of the population with simplified "products" (i.e., concepts) based on educational messages for behavior change (Lefebvre and Flora, 1988). In the United States and other Western countries, social marketing has been used for antismoking campaigns as well as to promote physical activity, to reduce levels of cardiovascular disease, and to prevent substance abuse.

Social marketing strategies have shown promising results in encouraging exercise, improving diet, and addressing substance misuse (Gordon et al., 2006). The LEAN (Low-fat Eating for America Now) national social marketing campaign of the Kaiser Family Foundation demonstrated that successful social marketing efforts are built on scientific consensus and include a broad range of partners from the public and private sectors as well as professional associations based on collaborative agreements (Samuels,

---

[1] Psychographics is "market research or statistics classifying population groups according to psychological variables (as attitudes, values or fears)." See http://www.merriam-webster.com/dictionary/psychographics (accessed May 21, 2012).

1993). Although necessary to trigger community transformation processes, social marketing, awareness raising, and attitude change by themselves have long been recognized as insufficient to induce changes in most segments of the population (Green, 1970a). More comprehensive strategies are needed to address the various barriers to, and enablers of, behavioral and social changes.

Health Promotion

Health promotion approaches are different from social marketing approaches in that they engage people and organizations in the transformation process and that this engagement in the process constitutes in itself a desired change. Health promotion conceptualizes health as a product of everyday living and proposes values and principles for public health practice (Breslow, 1999; Kickbusch, 2003; Potvin and Jones, 2011). These values are outlined in the Ottawa Charter for Health Promotion as the basis for strategies to promote health and well-being through the reorientation of health services, healthy public policy and intersectoral action, community action, the development of personal skills, and the creation of healthy environments (WHO, 1986). While improved health and well-being are goals of health promotion, the guiding principles for health promotion initiatives are that they should be "empowering, participatory, holistic, intersectoral, equitable, sustainable, and multi-strategy" (Rootman et al., 2001).

The goals of health promotion initiatives are generally defined in terms of increasing the capacity of individuals and communities to control of their health and its determinants (Nutbeam, 1998b). Health promotion outcomes include health literacy, social action and mobilization, organizational change, and healthy public policy. These outcomes are viewed as having their own intrinsic value as well as being instrumental in achieving intermediate health outcomes and, ultimately, broader health and social outcomes (Nutbeam, 1998a).

Policy Change

The final approach involves changing the public policies that govern the lives of citizens in a given jurisdiction. Public policies are broadly defined by actions taken by a government in the pursuit of its vision of the public good. Policies are "the whole set of solutions initiated by public authorities" (Bernier and Clavier, 2011). Public policy occurs at various levels of jurisdiction—local, regional or state, national, and global—and it can take various forms. The report *Promoting Health: Intervention Strategies from Social and Behavioral Research* (IOM, 2000b) proposes five types of action through which governing bodies can use laws and policy to achieve health and safety. The first is to use taxation to create economic incentives and disincentives intended to shape consumers' behaviors. Examples include taxes on products such as tobacco or alcohol (e.g., Elder et al., 2010; Hopkins, 2001; Hopkins et al., 2001; Task Force on Community Preventive Services, 2005).

The second type of action is to influence norms and values through the informational environment, using social marketing as a strategy. This is often a first step in a progression toward full regulation. Social marketing campaigns on the benefits of seat-belt use paved the way for the enactment of direct regulation to impose sanctions on car passengers who did not buckle up. As such regulatory measures came into being, their enforcement with highway spot checks of seat-belt wearing was enhanced in its effectiveness by mass media publicity about the citations and fines being given for failure to have seat belts fastened (Vasudevan et al., 2009).

The third type of action is direct regulation of specific risky behaviors that makes those behaviors unlawful and penalizes them, for example laws prohibiting the use of cell phones while driving or smoking by individuals under age 18.

Fourth, indirect regulation consists of "actions taken by legislatures and administrative agencies to prevent injury or disease or to promote public health" (IOM, 2000b, p. 398). An example is the addition of fluoride to water to prevent dental caries.

The fifth type of action, deregulation, is the alleviation of laws in the interest of the public's health. For example, laws prohibiting bicycles on some roadways could be repealed if bike paths and sidewalks were constructed on those roadways, thereby facilitating more physical activity and less pollution.

Once one recognizes that many determinants of health are outside the health sector and that those determinants can be influenced by policy, influencing the content and process of public policy becomes a strategy for promoting health and wellness. This is especially true at the community level. For example, to challenge industry practices it is generally easier to pass local ordinances than to enact legislation at the state or national level, where legislative proposals can more readily be challenged by industry lobbies.

A public policy is much more than a document or a given piece of legislation (Bernier and Clavier, 2011). It is a product of the interplay between political actors and citizens who use their power and resources to influence the process of setting the policy agenda, defining the policy content, and mobilizing resources for its implementation (Hassenteufel, 2008). Policy making is thus best conceived of as a dynamic process that involves a spectrum of stages in iterative cycles: agenda setting, policy formulation, decision making, policy implementation, and policy evaluation (Howlett et al., 2009; Ottoson et al., 2009). Various opportunities to influence the policy process present themselves at various stages in the cycle. Public health enters the agenda-setting stage of the public policy process, linking products or living conditions to health outcomes.

The long evolution in tobacco legislation throughout the second half of the 20th century offers an example of all the different policy approaches used together. Starting with the scientific recognition of the negative health impact of tobacco smoking in a public health report in 1964, and moving to various bans on tobacco in public places and increasing taxes on tobacco products, the history of tobacco policy in Western countries has shown that even in the face of valid scientific evidence, influencing the policy-making process is a work of advocacy and political influence, building coalitions, staging the public debate, evaluating comprehensive statewide and community policies and programs, and disseminating the findings of those evaluations to other jurisdictions (Bernier and Clavier, 2011; Breton et al., 2008; Eriksen et al., 2007). Studies of the policy process have shown that such efforts require resources and work because the political arena is occupied by powerful actors who promote and finance divergent interests and because scientific evidence alone is insufficient. People have to understand it, be persuaded by it, and change their thinking to incorporate it.

Recognizing that many determinants of health are the responsibility of sectors of public administration other than health, the Health in All Policies project aims to equip public health practitioners with a rationale to partner with other sectors in the pursuit of a variety of policy objectives that do not directly affect health but whose impact on the determinants of health is well documented (WHO, 2010). A case in point is the advocacy role of public health for urban planning models that create more opportunities for active transportation under the rationale that any commuting strategy that does not involve the use of a car increases the daily level of physical activity. Other examples may be found in the 2011 IOM report *For the Public's Health: Revitalizing Law and Policy to Meet New Challenges*.

MODELS

The following section contains brief descriptions of four models of program planning, implementation, and evaluation. These models are offered as illustrative examples of various conceptual and organizational frameworks used in the field of community-based prevention. The first model, PRECEDE–PROCEED, differs from the others in that it also contains a decision-making component. For this reason, the PRECEDE–PROCEED model is also discussed in Chapter 4. The other three models in this section are used by planners to implement changes after needs have been assessed and priorities established. These models are not used for valuing or choosing between interventions.

PRECEDE–PROCEED

The PRECEDE–PROCEED is a planning and evaluation model that evolved over more than four decades and four book editions (Green and Kreuter, 2005). Initially designed as a health education model, PRECEDE–PROCEED currently integrates several strategies to transform the ecosystem of individual well-being. Elements of the ecosystem that are amenable to transformation are the environment, health, lifestyle, and quality of life (Figure 2-2). A mix of educational, advocacy, policy, regulatory, resource-mobilizing, and organizational strategies are used to modify the predisposing, reinforcing, and enabling factors of the ecosystem. This model has been widely used in planning and evaluating community- and settings-based health programs (see http://www.lgreen.net/bibliography.html).

Other models such as MATCH (Multilevel Approach Toward Community Health; Simons-Morton et al., 1988c), PATCH (Planned Approach to Community Health) from the Centers for Disease Control and Prevention (HHS, no date; Kreuter et al., 1997), and intervention mapping (Bartholomew et al., 2001) also build on and extend the PRECEDE–PROCEED model with the provision of federal and state consultation processes and more detailed mapping of theory onto interventions.

The Multilevel Approaches Toward Community Health Model

The Multilevel Approaches Toward Community Health (MATCH) model (Figure 2-3) provides a representation of the ecological levels in conjunction with the planning, implementation, and evaluation stages of a community organization process.

The MATCH model was developed by Simons-Morton and colleagues (Simons-Morton et al., 1988a,b,c, 1989, 1991, 1995) for the Centers for Disease Control and Prevention for use in intervention handbooks to assist communities in the planning and evaluation of community programs. It is an intervention model aimed at influencing health at three levels: individual, organizational, and governmental. Its developers characterize MATCH as an "organizing framework" designed to be applied after risk factors and priorities for action have been identified (Simons-Morton et al., 1988c).

The model originally consisted of four phases: health goals selection, intervention planning, implementation, and evaluation. Each phase has multiple components that give the model the flexibility to be adapted to the context of the target population, community, or intervention. It can be used for a variety of interventions, from strategies to improve hypertension medication compliance to population-level interventions aimed at preventing injuries, such as programs to increase seat-belt use.

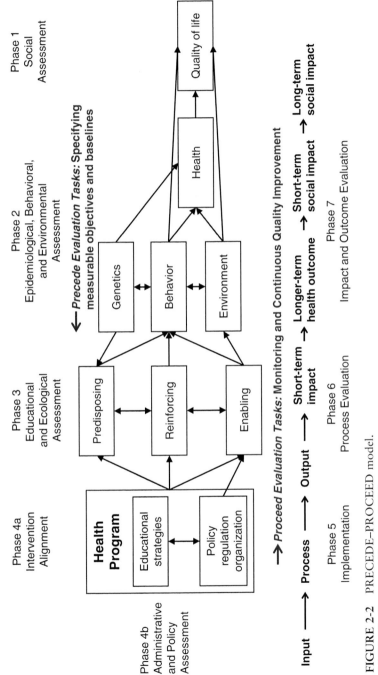

FIGURE 2-2 PRECEDE–PROCEED model.
SOURCE: Green and Kreuter, 2005.

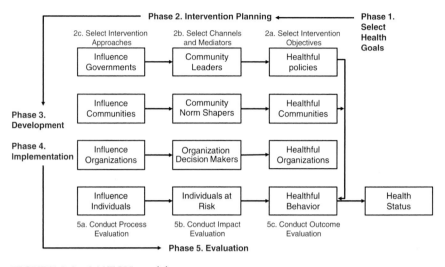

FIGURE 2-3 MATCH model.
SOURCE: Simons-Morton et al., 1995.

The selection of health goals can be based on a number of factors, ranging from epidemiological data to community preference or the personal interest of an individual. The second and third phases, intervention planning and implementation, can be targeted at either the individuals or communities whose health is affected or at those whose funding or policy decisions affect these individuals or communities. Each intervention has varying approaches and intensities and can therefore be tailored to the needs of the target group. Finally, the intervention is evaluated based on process, impact, and outcome. The evaluation determines whether the intervention led to progress toward the health goals identified in the first phase. This includes, in the case of the interventions aimed at organizations or governments, whether the intervention led to other interventions (Simons-Morton, 1988).

The Swiss Model for Outcome Classification in Health Promotion and Prevention

The Swiss Model for Outcome Classification in Health Promotion and Prevention (SMOC) is a planning and evaluation tool developed by Health Promotion Switzerland and the Institutes for Social and Preventive Medicine in Bern and Lausanne to aid in health promotion efforts. The model is intended to be broadly applied and to provide an overview of activities for planners and evaluators. It also establishes a common language to ease communication among stakeholders, and it helps with determining objectives and indicators. Originally developed for use with individual projects, SMOC has also proven useful for higher-level planning (Spencer et al., 2008).

The SMOC model is based on the work of Nutbeam (2000), which presented an outcome model for health promotion activities (Nutbeam, 2000; Spencer et al., 2008). The Nutbeam model moves from health promotion actions through health promotion outcomes and intermediate health outcomes to health and social outcomes measured by, among other things, morbidity, mortality, and disability. Nutbeam attempts to provide a bridge between the intervention and its goals, listing potential measures of progress between the two (Nutbeam, 2000).

SMOC (Figure 2-4) builds on this concept. It contains four levels: health promotion measures (A), factors influencing health determinants (B), health determinants (C), and health status (D). Within the four levels are 16 categories that provide further detail and guidance to users of the model. It is important to note that there are no arrows in the model. Although it is clear that each level has an impact on the subsequent level, the lack of arrows acknowledges that each level or category can provide feedback or have an effect on any other part of the process without the sequence of effects necessarily being linear. This flexibility is intended to make the model adaptable in dealing with real world situations and a wide range of stakeholders (Spencer et al., 2008).

The Community Development Model

The community development model includes three important concepts: decentralization, participatory planning and implementation of programs, and multisectoral involvement. Ideally, decentralization places the planning and evaluation functions at the local level and keeps the highly specialized resources, including expensive technology and facilities, at the central level. The effective delivery of community development programs necessarily depends on both central and local organizations.

The participatory planning and implementation aspect of the model, which applies both to organizations and individuals, involves people in an affected community setting their own priorities and goals and planning out programs that will serve them. Expecting neighborhoods and organizations to implement programs planned elsewhere often yields only limited local commitment to the goals and methods of the program (Bracht, 1998; Rothman and Brown, 1989). Efforts that involve community participation often require a longer time for planning and coordination because of the need to enlist the cooperation and participation of members of the community (Green, 1986a,b).

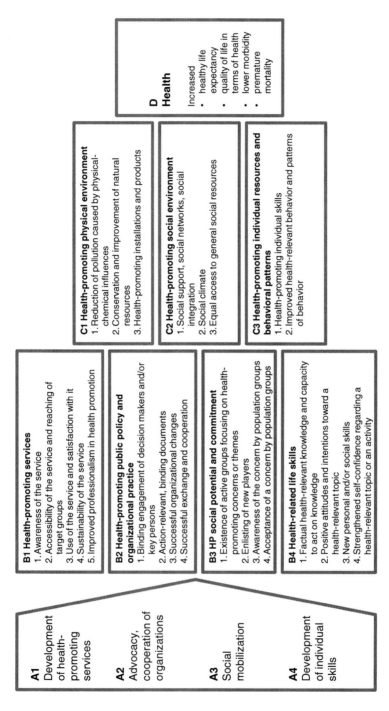

A1
Development of health-promoting services

A2
Advocacy, cooperation of organizations

A3
Social mobilization

A4
Development of individual skills

B1 Health-promoting services
1. Awareness of the service
2. Accessibility of the service and reaching of target groups
3. Use of the service and satisfaction with it
4. Sustainability of the service
5. Improved professionalism in health promotion

B2 Health-promoting public policy and organizational practice
1. Binding engagement of decision makers and/or key persons
2. Action-relevant, binding documents
3. Successful organizational changes
4. Successful exchange and cooperation

B3 HP social potential and commitment
1. Existence of active groups focusing on health-promoting concerns or themes
2. Enlisting of new players
3. Awareness of the concern by population groups
4. Acceptance of a concern by population groups

B4 Health-related life skills
1. Factual health-relevant knowledge and capacity to act on knowledge
2. Positive attitudes and intentions toward a health-relevant topic
3. New personal and/or social skills
4. Strengthened self-confidence regarding a health-relevant topic or an activity

C1 Health-promoting physical environment
1. Reduction of pollution caused by physical-chemical influences
2. Conservation and improvement of natural resources
3. Health-promoting installations and products

C2 Health-promoting social environment
1. Social support, social networks, social integration
2. Social climate
3. Equal access to general social resources

C3 Health-promoting individual resources and behavioral patterns
1. Health-promoting individual skills
2. Improved health-relevant behavior and patterns of behavior

D
Health

Increased
• healthy life expectancy
• quality of life in terms of health
• lower morbidity
• premature mortality

FIGURE 2-4 Overview of the Swiss Model for Outcome Classification in Health Promotion and Prevention.
SOURCE: Spencer et al., 2008.

Multisectoral involvement is the inclusion of representatives from a variety of sectors that can help effect change. Often such inclusion takes the form of a coalition, which might include representatives from recreation, business, media, and welfare sectors as well as from medical and health sectors. Coalitions have the value of bringing multiple stakeholders together to agree on goals and broad strategy. Many organizations outside the health field have taken up health-related programs because they perceive a public demand for health promotion, better health protection, or health service. Commercial interests, in particular, have risen to the challenge of consumer demand. As Kickbusch and Payne (2003) observed, "[I]n the United States alone the sales of the wellness industry have already reached approximately $200 billion, and it is set to achieve sales of $1 trillion within 10 years."

The community development model has been widely applied, albeit with varying success. Pilot projects in Toronto and California inspired the Healthy Communities efforts in both Canada and the United States. The World Health Organization promoted the Healthy Cities movement to encourage city governments to take a broad, multisectoral approach to planning for health promotion. Underlying the approach is the ecological model discussed earlier, that is, a broad view of the determinants of health, including policies and environmental conditions that influence the health of whole populations. The community development model emphasizes the disparities in health and the need for more equitable distribution of health-related resources to close the gaps between subpopulations.

Recent applications of the community development model in Australia, Europe, and Canada have been carried out under the Healthy Cities and Healthy Communities initiatives (Inayatullah, 2011; Larsen and Manderson, 2009). In the United States, community development in health has occurred under the Planned Approach to Community Health (PATCH) model. PATCH was first developed by the Centers for Disease Control and Prevention (CDC) in 1983 as a way of reconciling federal funding requirements, which were locked into specific disease categories, with the community development principles of local planning for needs that communities themselves identify. The designers of PATCH based their approach on the traditions of state and community capacity-building and data-based planning and monitoring of programs. The PRECEDE–PROCEED model of planning and evaluation along with community development principles of local ownership were applied in PATCH (Green and Kreuter, 1992). By 1987, 25 PATCH programs had been initiated in 12 states, and by 1997 several hundred were under way across the United States (Kreuter, 1992). Dozens more programs were modeled after this approach in Australia, Canada, China, and Europe.

IMPACT OF COMMUNITY-BASED PREVENTION

As discussed earlier, community-based prevention can involve complex systems of coordinated actions which include numerous actors, many acting in concert through organizational partnerships and coalitions. Ideally the partnerships include intersectoral collaboration between health organizations and their public-sector counterparts in education, social services, and city planning as well as private-sector business interests that influence the diets, physical activity, tobacco consumption, and other behaviors of the public that affect health. Evaluation seeks to determine the effectiveness of these efforts; it poses many methodological and practical problems because of the complex and systemic nature of community-based prevention (Mercer et al., 2007).

A frequently cited example of community-based prevention is the North Karelia study in Finland (Puska and Uutela, 2000; Puska et al., 1985, 1998). This was a grassroots initiative, begun in 1972, aimed at reducing the community's high rates of death from coronary heart disease (the highest in the world at that time). Local authorities consulted with and received technical assistance from researchers in formulating and implementing the project. Initially, the main focus was improving dietary habits and reducing rates of smoking, but these goals were later enlarged to include the broader objectives of chronic disease prevention and health promotion in both children and adults. Box 2-1 provides a summary of the project's achievements.

Key features of the program were

- a carefully outlined theoretical framework;
- community involvement;
- a flexible and dynamic intervention, adapting to naturally occurring events;
- a multifaceted intervention, including innovative media campaigns, health care providers, environmental changes, and industry and policy changes; and
- strong leadership and institutional support.

The North Karelia project inspired efforts sponsored by the National Institutes of Health to implement and evaluate similar community interventions in California with the Stanford Three-Community and the Stanford Five-Community studies. In a series of commentaries and editorials published following the release of disappointing results, leading epidemiologists acknowledged the limitations of the controlled experiment to assess the value of such interventions on a community scale (Fisher, 1995; Fortmann et al., 1995; Suser, 1995; Winkleby, 1994; Winkleby et al., 1996).

BOX 2-1
Achievements of the North Karelia Project: 2005/2007

Smoking rates decreased from 52 percent to 31 percent in men, although the rates increased from 10 percent to 18 percent in women.

Mean serum cholesterol (mmol/L) decreased from 6.9 to 5.4 in men (a 21 percent drop) and from 6.8 to 5.2 in women (a 23 percent drop).

Mean blood pressure (mmHg) decreased from 149/92 to 139/83 in men and from 153/92 to 134/78 in women.

Reductions in age-adjusted mortality for men, 35-64 years of age, between 1970 and 1995:

- All causes: 63 percent
- All cardiovascular causes: 80 percent
- Coronary heart disease: 85 percent (this is the most rapid decline in the world to date)
- All cancers: 67 percent
- Lung cancer: 71 percent (1997)

SOURCES: Puska and Uutela, 2000; Puska et al., 2009.

The 9-year Stanford project did show that the blood pressure improvements observed in all cities from baseline to the end of the intervention were maintained during the follow-up in treatment cities but not in control cities. Cholesterol levels continued to decline in all cities during follow-up. Smoking rates leveled out or increased slightly in treatment cities and continued to decline in control cities, but the differences were not significant. Both coronary heart disease and all-cause mortality risk scores were maintained or continued to improve in treatment cities while leveling out or going back up in control cities (Winkleby et al., 1996).

Reviews by the Task Force on Community Preventive Services as well as the Cochrane reviews have synthesized evidence concerning community prevention efforts. Such syntheses give somewhat mixed results concerning the effectiveness of the interventions. They are useful, however, in providing examples of implementation approaches for community-based prevention. For example, Brinn and colleagues (2010) examined the impact of media and multi-component campaigns to prevent youth from starting to smoke. They identified a total of 84 published evaluations reporting on media campaigns. Unfortunately, only seven of those were conducted using some form of control groups, randomized or not, including time series in which groups were used as their own control with a sufficiently long pre-intervention period and number of observations. Only three of those studies found the campaign to have helped prevent smoking among people aged 25 years and younger. The effective campaigns were conducted in combination with some school educational activities and used messages developed through extensive formative evaluation. A Cochrane review of multi-component tobacco prevention programs found only 25 controlled trials, only 9 of which reported significant long-term reductions in smoking (Carson et al., 2011).

Among other community interventions, a review of non-legislative interventions to increase bicycle helmet use in children identified four community-based interventions that positively affected helmet use (Owen et al., 2011). Components of the interventions included subsidized helmets, local media campaigns, and helmet education programs. Similarly, in a review of 25 community trials to prevent the uptake of tobacco smoking by youth, Carson and colleagues (2011), identified 10 studies with a significant positive outcome. All successful interventions included a mix of complementary interventions taking place in various community settings, including schools and media campaigns.

The Community Guide to Preventive Services (also known as the Community Guide [www.thecommunityguide.org]) uses systematic, objective, and consistent methods to evaluate evidence for the effectiveness for certain interventions or categories of interventions. Where possible, the Community Guide also reviews evidence of the economic efficiency of the intervention (Briss et al., 2004). An economic evaluation of home-based asthma interventions with an environmental focus was conducted using the methods developed for the Community Guide. For the 13 studies included in the evaluation, the annual total program costs per participant ranged from $231 to $14,858 (in 2007 dollars), depending on the level of environmental remediation carried out in the intervention. Of the 13 studies, annual medical costs averted per participant could be calculated for 6 of them; those annual costs averted ranged from $147 to $10,093 per person. It was possible to calculate incremental cost effectiveness ratios (ICER) for only three of the studies; these ranged from $12 to $57 per symptom-free day (Nurmagambetov et al., 2011). Based on this the Community Preventive Services Task Force found that "home-based, multi-trigger, multicomponent interventions with a combination of minor or moderate environmental remediation with an educational component provide good value for the money invested" (see www.thecommunityguide.org/asthma/multicomponent.html).

Three worksite programs to prevent and control obesity reported cost-effectiveness numbers that ranged from $1.44 to $4.16 per pound of weight loss (Anderson et al., 2009). The use of cost-effectiveness per pound of weight loss is an example of the sort of intermediate outcomes that need to be identified in any study that, like this one, is aiming at a very long-term goal (in this case, the prevention of obesity). A review of diabetes self-management education (DSME) programs completed in 2002 found that there was sufficient evidence of effectiveness to recommend DSME programs be implemented in community gathering places for adults with type 2 diabetes. (Norris et al., 2002) At that time, no studies were found that would permit an economic evaluation of these programs (see http://www.thecommunityguide.org/diabetes/selfmgeducation.html).

In 2011 Thorpe and colleagues estimated that enrolling individuals aged 60-64 who are prediabetic in the YMCA's community-based diabetes prevention program could save Medicare between $1.8 billion and $2.3 billion over 10 years by averting future medical costs of diabetes in this population (Thorpe and Yang, 2011). Another study that examined Medicare costs between 1997 and 2006 found that the costs were increasing more rapidly for obese Medicare recipients than for those with normal weight (Alley et al., 2012). Finkelstein and colleagues (2009) found that medical costs were higher for obese individuals and that those costs were increasing. They estimated that the rise in obesity prevalence accounted for 89 percent of the increase in obesity spending between 1998 and 2006 (Finkelstein et al., 2009).

Bradley and colleagues (2011) analyzed data on spending for health and social services for member countries in the Organisation for Economic Co-operation and Development (OECD). They found that greater spending on social services such as anti-poverty programs, employment programs, and housing support was significantly associated with increased life expectancy, decreased infant mortality, and decreased potential years of life lost. This suggests that there is a link between programs that address the social determinants of poor health and improved population health. Within the OECD, the United States spends nearly twice as much on health care—measured as a percentage of GDP—than other countries, but it ranks in the bottom third in key population health indicators such as life expectancy and infant and maternal mortality (Bradley et al., 2011).

EVALUATION OF COMMUNITY-BASED PREVENTION

For the past 15 years there has been a lively debate in the scientific community about the pros and cons of experimental and observational methods for the evaluation of community interventions (Mercer et al., 2007; Potvin and Richard, 2001). A major issue in evaluating community-based interventions concerns the role of context. The experimental paradigm supposes that interventions are exogenous, that is, that a part of the stimulus and at least some of the support comes from outside of the community and is not created by it. Such exogenous intervention components may take various forms, such as resources (money from a foundation or a federal funding program), knowledge (professional expertise, scientific report, professional practice guidelines based on systematic reviews of evidence), or technical devices (written curriculum, processed food). Nevertheless, research has shown that to have an effect those external resources must have cultural relevance and to be adapted to local conditions (Tirodkar et al., 2010). Thus the randomized controlled trial that requires a consistent protocol of replication and emphasizes the importance of internal validity (causal certainty) is difficult to use in evaluating community-based prevention interventions.

Another problem for replicability is that the effectiveness of a community intervention is not inherent within the intervention itself (that is, within what is imported from outside). Rather, its effectiveness lies in the interaction between the intervention and the contextual conditions. As a consequence, the actual events and actions that form an intervention in context will differ across various settings, even if the external part of this intervention is held constant (Hawe et al., 2004).

This state of affairs raises a variety of issues from an experimental perspective that presupposes that contextual conditions are controlled for. Even when it is possible to identify objectively the exogenous component of the intervention, systematic observations are needed in order to trace and model the multiple transformations and adaptations such components must go through in order to produce the observable set of unique actions and their impact that characterize a given program. The Kaiser Family Foundation grants program in the 1990s provides an interesting example of a trial that sought to document these interactions between the exogenous components and the community contexts (Wagner et al., 2000). Eleven communities were randomized among qualified applicants to receive funding for a period of 5 years to identify their health needs and develop action plans. Health needs covered a wide range of issues. Community activation was conceived of as an intermediary mechanism that would, because of the activities funded in the selected communities, be elevated compared to a set of 11 comparable communities that did not receive external funding. Results were disappointing, however, as there was no observed difference in community activation between funded and not-funded communities. In terms of health outcomes, results varied and only marginally significant effects were observed for some dietary behaviors in some of the funded communities (Wagner et al., 2000).

This study and another conducted by Hallfors et al. (2002) raise two questions. First, does the outside funding used to initiate a community-organization and coalition-development process create artificial conditions of coalition formation that undercut the effectiveness often attributed to community-initiated coalitions that are not externally initiated (Green and Kreuter, 2002)? Second, might the requirement of outside funding agencies mandating participation through coalitions of multiple organizations rather than through partnerships of a smaller number be a potential detriment to effective community initiative (Green, 2000)?

Changes in communities take time, and for such changes to affect the health of residents it takes even more time. The more distal the targeted risk factors to the health outcome, the more time is required for the intervention to produce effect (de Leeuw, 2011; El Ansari et al., 2001). In addition to the feasibility problems of following communities and (mobile) populations for long periods of time, the long-term nature of community intervention effects makes them more susceptible to interacting with other interventions or historical events, blurring or even dissipating their effect. Researchers and evaluators in health promotion have addressed this problem by creating models of intermediary impact that logically link the intervention to ultimate health and wellness impact (e.g., the models described in this chapter and Chapter 4 and the findings and recommendations of the Task Force on Community Preventive Services [http://www.thecommunityguide.org]). These models provide theoretical intermediary checkpoints to assess the direction of changes (if any) associated with the intervention.

In evaluating a community intervention it is critical to be able to link process and outcome evaluation in order to understand how the exogenous components of an intervention interact with local conditions. Such a linking serves the dual purpose of understanding the local adaptations that necessarily take place and of documenting how such programs evolve. Indeed, if interventions are responsive to environmental conditions, it follows that effective interventions will involve and change in response to the changes they produce in community context. Such a dynamic process can only be captured through systematic observations informed by strong theoretical models of change.

Much progress has been made in the conceptualization of community interventions over the past 50 years. One recognized success is in tobacco control (Box 2-2). The science of community intervention is very young and, compared to the historically successful basic sciences, the knowledge base upon which action can be founded contains numerous gaps. The links between the various observations compiled are still very speculative. This is why it is so important to include research and evaluation components in any community-based intervention. Such research is needed to better understand how community interventions work. There exist only a few initiatives worldwide that propose to synthesize the results of evaluations of community-based prevention strategies and wellness policy, including the Cochrane review groups on population and public health, and the CDC-facilitated work of the Task Force on Community Preventive Services.

The Need for More Research and Novel Paradigms

While a few community-based prevention interventions have passed the Community Guide standards for using appropriate methodology for

---

BOX 2-2
The Case of Tobacco Control Policies as a Template
for Successful Community Health Change

Policies and programs work better when they are interdependent and synergistic, as demonstrated by the CDC's Office on Smoking and Health (1999, 2007) and others that have concluded from the successes of statewide and community tobacco control programs that comprehensive tobacco control must coordinate policies and programs that depend on each other for success. Such programs and policies emanate from different levels of organizations and government, and each component reaches different segments of the population. For example, states cannot reach effectively into local organizations, and localities cannot afford the cost of mass media placements.

An informed and concerned public makes it easier to introduce new policies (Green and Richard, 1993). Informational, educational, and motivational messages through various media and channels facilitate awareness and concern. For youth there is a need for mass media to provide a backdrop of messages and images that are consistent with those they receive from family, teachers, and programs. Hollywood film images of smokers who are protagonists and magazine advertisements with images of glamorous models smoking, for example, send an inconsistent message about smoking from those presented in tobacco-cessation programs.

The tobacco industry outspends state tobacco control programs at least $10 to $1, and up to 20 to 1 on media and marketing during political campaigns to raise taxes on cigarettes (Begay et al., 1993; Pierce and Gilpin, 2004; Tobacco Education and Research Oversight Committee, 2009; Traynor et al., 1993). In the 1970s most political efforts at state and federal levels to ban smoking in public places were successfully beaten back by tobacco industry, but most city and county initiatives to regulate smoking during that same period passed because the industry could not put out the multiplicity of brush fires at the local level (NCI, 2000). Coordinating local and state policy and program efforts has been key to the notable successes of California and other states and municipalities in smoking-cessation efforts (Best et al., 2007; Tobacco Education and Research Oversight Committee, 2009). When each level of government and voluntary agency action coordinates and divides the labor of comprehensive programs and policies, the synergy produces more successful outcomes.

---

evaluation, many community-based interventions are implemented without adequate evaluation. This has resulted in a scarcity of information about the effectiveness of these interventions. A number of factors have been identified to explain this relative scarcity, including the small number of evaluations undertaken (as mentioned above), methodological difficulties, and a lack of theoretical clarity.

One set of factors is related to the fact that few interventions are rigorously evaluated, relative to the number of past and ongoing efforts in communities across many countries. There are many more or less defined interventions being implemented by various actors in a community with various levels of resource investments. Most of these interventions are unknown to all except those directly involved. For example, Spinks et al. (2009) commented that, despite the identification of more than 200 communities worldwide with a WHO Safe Community status, only a handful in two regions of the world have been subject to controlled evaluation. If little is known, it is partly because the issue has not been widely studied.

Another set of factors relates to methodology. Randomized controlled trials, the gold standard in clinical medicine, have proven difficult to undertake for the evaluation of community-based interventions. As discussed earlier, randomized controlled trials require adherence to a set protocol, yet a key characteristic of community-based prevention is to make sure that the intervention is tailored to the affected community, usually with significant input from community members themselves. Such adjustment in the intervention makes it difficult to identify control communities for comparison purposes.

In addition to these methodological difficulties, there might also be a lack of theoretical clarity about the effective mechanisms operating in such interventions and the full range of potential effects that might be influenced by these interventions (Hawe et al., 2004).

Communities have long histories, and their composition in terms of both population characteristics and structural elements is not conducive to rapid change (De Koninck and Pampalon, 2007). Changing the course of such systems is a long-term endeavor and requires a locally valid model of the possible pathways through which such transformations can be spearheaded. Evaluating non-standardized, constantly changing, community-directed, slow-moving changes at all the levels in ecological models from programs to policies presents methodological, logistical, and economic feasibility challenges. It is impossible to determine the relative contributions of all the many moving parts or the active ingredients in the complex interventions (Mercer et al., 2007). Deconstructing complex interventions may not even be advisable, given that ecological models guiding the projects emphasize the need for multi-level interventions and the reciprocal dependency of many of the interventions and policies (Sallis et al., 2008).

The strategic vision of the Office of Behavioral and Social Sciences Research (OBSSR) at the National Institutes of Health recognizes that prevailing paradigms focusing on single-cause, single-discipline, and single-level-of-analysis models are necessary but insufficient and calls for interdisciplinary and multilevel approaches that integrate biological, behavioral, and social sciences to address the complex issues that challenge the public's health (Mabry et al., 2008). Furthermore, the prevailing linear research-to-practice paradigms, while useful for addressing specific clinical or epidemiologic questions, are often inadequate to tackle real-world health problems that are intrinsically imbedded in the widely varying complexities of behavioral, social, and cultural settings (Livingood et al., 2011).

As with the earlier academically directed intervention studies, however, even when considering these complexities, evaluations of community-based programs, policies, and strategies cannot assure that an effective intervention in one setting will generalize to another community. Emerging paradigms call for the integration of research and practice, similar to the integrations in applied physical sciences, engineering, and architecture (Livingood et al., 2011). These approaches represent a radical departure from best practice interventions and involve the customization of scientific principles and methods to each situation. They offer a greater degree of credibility about their generalizability insofar as they are carried out in real time by real practitioners and community partners (Green, 2007).

The following chapter examines system thinking in greater detail, describing how systems science can be used to explore the complexity of community-based prevention. That chapter also discusses domains of value for community-based prevention interventions.

REFERENCES

Adler, N., A. Singh-Manoux, J. Schwartz, J. Stewart, K. Matthews, and M. G. Marmot. 2008. Social status and health: A comparison of British civil servants in Whitehall II with European- and African-Americans in CARDIA. *Social Science and Medicine* 66(5):1034-1045.

Alley, D., J. Lloyd, T. Shaffer, and B. Stuart. 2012. Changes in the association between body mass index and Medicare costs, 1997-2006. *Archives of Internal Medicine* 172(3):277.

Anderson, L. M., T. A. Quinn, K. Glanz, G. Ramirez, L. C. Kahwati, D. B. Johnson, L. R. Buchanan, W. R. Archer, S. Chattopadhyay, and G. P. Kalra. 2009. The effectiveness of worksite nutrition and physical activity interventions for controlling employee overweight and obesity: A systematic review. *American Journal of Preventive Medicine* 37(4):340-357.

Antonovsky, A. 1967. Social class, life expectancy and overall mortality. *Milbank Memorial Fund Quarterly* 45(2):31-73.

Bartholomew, L. K., G. S. Parcel, G. Kok, and N. H. Gottlieb. 2001. *Intervention mapping: Designing theory- and evidence-based health promotion programs*. Mountain View, CA: McGraw-Hill.

Becker, M. H. 1974. *The health belief model and personal health behavior*. Thorofare, NJ: Slack, Inc.

Begay, M. E., M. Traynor, and S. A. Glantz. 1993. The tobacco industry, state politics, and tobacco education in California. *American Journal of Public Health* 83(9):1214-1221.

Berkman, L., and T. A. Glass. 2000. Social integration, social networks, social support, and health. In *Social epidemiology*, edited by L. Berkman and I. Kawachi. New York: Oxford University Press. Pp. 137-173.

Berkman, L., and I. Kawachi. 2000. *Social epidemiology*. New York: Oxford University Press.

Bernier, N. F., and C. Clavier. 2011. Public health policy research: Making the case for a political science approach. *Health Promotion International* 26(1):109-116.

Best, A., P. I. Clark, S. J. Leischow, and W. Trochim. 2007. *Greater than the sum: Systems thinking in tobacco control.* Bethesda, MD: National Institutes of Health.

Bleich, S. N., M. P. Jarlenski, C. N. Bell, and T. A. Laveist. 2011. Health inequalities: Trends, progress, and policy. *Annual Review of Public Health* 33:7-40.

Bracht, N. F. 1998. *Health promotion at the community level: New advances*, 2nd Ed. New York: Sage.

Bradley, E. H., B. R. Elkins, J. Herrin, and B. Elbel. 2011. Health and social services expenditures: Associations with health outcomes. *BMJ Quality and Safety* 20(10):826-831.

Brennan, L. K. 2002. *Community perceptions and physical activity: An examination of the correspondence between protective social factors and behavior.* St. Louis, MO: Saint Louis University.

Breslow, L. 1999. From disease prevention to health promotion. *JAMA* 281(11):1030-1033.

Breton, E., L. Richard, F. Gagnon, M. Jacques, and P. Bergeron. 2008. Health promotion research and practice require sound policy analysis models: The case of Quebec's tobacco act. *Social Science and Medicine* 67(11):1679-1689.

Brinn, M. P., K. V. Carson, A. J. Esterman, A. B. Chang, and B. J. Smith. 2010. Mass media interventions for preventing smoking in young people. *Cochrane Database of Systematic Reviews* 11:CD001006.

Briss, P., B. Rimer, B. Reilley, R. C. Coates, N. C. Lee, P. Mullen, P. Corso, A. B. Hutchinson, R. Hiatt, J. Kerner, P. George, C. White, N. Gandhi, M. Saraiya, R. Breslow, G. Isham, S. M. Teutsch, A. R. Hinman, and R. Lawrence. 2004. Promoting informed decisions about cancer screening in communities and healthcare systems. *American Journal of Preventive Medicine* 26(1):67-80.

Brownson, R. C., E. K. Proctor, and G. A. Colditz. 2012. *Dissemination and implimentation science.* New York: Oxford University Press.

Cargo, M., and S. L. Mercer. 2008. The value and challenges of participatory research: Strengthening its practice. *Annual Review of Public Health* 29:325-350.

Carson, K. V., M. P. Brinn, N. A. Labiszewski, A. J. Esterman, A. B. Chang, and B. J. Smith. 2011. Community interventions for preventing smoking in young people. *Cochrane Database of Systematic Reviews* 7:CD001291.

Cheadle, A., W. Beery, E. Wagner, S. Fawcett, L. Green, D. Moss, A. Plough, A. Wandersman, and I. Woods. 1997. Conference report: Community-based health promotion—state of the art and recommendations for the future. *American Journal of Preventive Medicine* 13(4):240.

Cockerham, W. C., A. Rütten, and T. Abel. 1997. Conceptualizing contemporary health lifestyles. *Sociological Quarterly* 38(2):321-342.

Cohen, S., I. Brissette, D. P. Skoner, and W. J. Doyle. 2000. Social integration and health: The case of the common cold. *Journal of Social Structure* 1(3):1-7.

Dahlgren, G., and M. Whitehead. 1991. *Policies and strategies to promote social equity in health.* Stockholm: Institute for Future Studies.

De Koninck, M., and R. Pampalon. 2007. Living environments and health at the local level: The case of three localities in the Québec city region. *Canadian Journal of Public Health* 98(Suppl 1):S45-S53.

de Leeuw, E. 2011. Do healthy cities work? A logic of method for assessing impact and outcome of healthy cities. *Journal of Urban Health* 89(2): 217-231.

Deasy, L. C. 1956. Socio-economic status and participation in the poliomyelitis vaccine trial. *American Sociological Review* 21(2):185-191.

Diehr, P., P. Hannon, B. Pizacani, M. Forehand, H. Meischke, S. Curry, D. P. Martin, M. R. Weaver, and J. Harris. 2011. Social marketing, stages of change, and public health smoking interventions. *Health Education and Behavior* 38(2):123-131.

D'Onofrio, C. N. 1966. *Reaching our hard to reach—the unvaccinated*. Berkeley, CA: California State Department of Public Health.

Donovan, R., N. Henley, and MyiLibrary Ltd. 2010. *Principles and practice of social marketing: An international perspective*. New York: Cambridge University Press.

Dressendorfer, R. H., K. Raine, R. J. Dyck, R. C. Plotnikoff, R. L. Collins-Nakai, W. K. McLaughlin, and K. Ness. 2005. A conceptual model of community capacity development for health promotion in the Alberta Heart Health Project. *Health Promotion Practice* 6(1):31-36.

Edmundo, K., W. Guimarães, M. do Socorro Vasconcelos, A. P. Baptista, and D. Becker. 2005. Network of communities in the fight against AIDS: Local actions to address health inequities and promote health in Rio de Janeiro, Brazil. *Promotion and Education* 12(3 Suppl):15-19.

El Ansari, W., C. J. Phillips, and M. Hammick. 2001. Collaboration and partnerships: Developing the evidence base. *Health and Social Care in the Community* 9(4):215-227.

Elder, R. W., B. Lawrence, A. Ferguson, T. S. Naimi, R. D. Brewer, S. K. Chattopadhyay, T. L. Toomey, and J. E. Fielding. 2010. The effectiveness of tax policy interventions for reducing excessive alcohol consumption and related harms. *American Journal of Preventive Medicine* 38(2):217-229.

Eller, M., R. Holle, R. Landgraf, and A. Mielck. 2008. Social network effect on self-rated health in type 2 diabetic patients—results from a longitudinal population-based study. *International Journal of Public Health* 53(4):188-194.

Eriksen, M. P., L. W. Green, C. G. Husten, L. L. Pederson, and T. F. Pechacek. 2007. Thank you for not smoking: The public health response to tobacco-related mortality in the United States. In *Silent victories: The history and practice of public health in twentieth-century America*, edited by J. W. Ward and C. S. Warren. New York: Oxford University Press. Pp. 423-436.

Evans, R. G., and G. L. Stoddart. 1990. Producing health, consuming health care. *Social Science Medicine* 31(12):1347-1363.

Finkelstein, E. A., J. G. Trogdon, J. W. Cohen, and W. Dietz. 2009. Annual medical spending attributable to obesity: Payer- and service-specific estimates. *Health Affairs* 28(5):w822-w831.

Fisher, E. B., Jr. 1995. The results of the COMMIT trial. Community intervention trial for smoking cessation. *American Journal of Public Health* 85(2):159-160.

Fortmann, S. P., J. A. Flora, M. A. Winkleby, C. Schooler, C. B. Taylor, and J. W. Farquhar. 1995. Community intervention trials: Reflections on the Stanford Five-City Project experience. *American Journal of Epidemiology* 142(6):576-586.

French, J. 2009. The nature, development and contribution of social marketing to public health practice since 2004 in England. *Perspectives in Public Health* 129(6):262-267.

Frohlich, K. L., E. Corin, and L. Potvin. 2001. A theoretical proposal for the relationship between context and disease. *Sociology of Health and Illness* 23(6):776-797.

Gauderman, W. J., E. Avol, F. Gilliland, H. Vora, D. Thomas, K. Berhane, R. McConnell, N. Kuenzli, F. Lurmann, and E. Rappaport. 2004. The effect of air pollution on lung development from 10 to 18 years of age. *New England Journal of Medicine* 351(11):1057-1067.

Gibson, L., J. Doherty, R. Loewnson, V. Francis, and WHO Health Systems Knowledge Network. 2007. *Challenging inequity through health systems: Final report of the health systems knowledge network*. Geneva: WHO Commission on the Social Determinants of Health.

Gordon, R., L. McDermott, M. Stead, and K. Angus. 2006. The effectiveness of social marketing interventions for health improvement: What's the evidence? *Public Health* 120(12):1133-1139.

Green, L. W. 1970a. Should health education abandon attitude change strategies? Perspectives from recent research. *Health Education Monographs* 30:25-48.

Green, L. W. 1970b. *Status identity and preventive health behavior.* Berkeley, CA: School of Public Health, University of California.

Green, L. W. 1986a. *New policies for health education in primary health care.* Geneva: World Health Organization.

Green, L. W. 1986b. The theory of participation: A qualitative analysis of its expression in national and international health policies. *Advances in Health Education and Promotion* 1:211-236.

Green, L. W. 2000. Caveats on coalitions: In praise of partnerships. *Health Promotion Practice* 1(1):64-65.

Green, L. W. 2007. Translation 2 research: The roadmap less traveled. *American Journal of Preventive Medicine* 33(2):137-138.

Green, L. W., and M. W. Kreuter. 1992. CDC's planned approach to community health as an application of Precede and an inspiration for Proceed. *Journal of Health Education* 23(3):140-147.

Green, L. W., and M. W. Kreuter. 2002. Fighting back or fighting themselves? Community coalitions against substance abuse and their use of best practices. *American Journal of Preventive Medicine* 23(4):303.

Green, L. W., and M. W. Kreuter. 2005. *Health program planning: An educational and ecological approach*, 4th ed. New York: McGraw-Hill.

Green, L. W., and A. L. McAlister. 1984. Macro-intervention to support health behavior: Some theoretical perspectives and practical reflections. *Health Education & Behavior* 11(3):323-339.

Green, L. W., and L. Richard. 1993. The need to combine health education and health promotion: The case of cardiovascular disease prevention. *Promotion and Education* Spec No:11-18.

Green, L. W., J. M. Ottoson, C. García, and R. A. Hiatt. 2009. Diffusion theory and knowledge dissemination, utilization, and integration in public health. *Annual Review of Public Health* 30(1):151-174.

Hackett, C. 1982. McLetchie on mass campaigns. *Tropical Doctor* 12(1):35-38.

Hallfors, D., H. Cho, D. Livert, and C. Kadushin. 2002. Fighting back against substance abuse: Are community coalitions winning? *American Journal of Preventive Medicine* 23(4):237-245.

Handy, S. 2004. *Community design and physical activity: What do we know? And what don't we know.* http://www.des.ucdavis.edu/faculty/handy/Handy_NIEHS_revised.pdf (accessed June 5, 2012).

Harrison, J. A., P. D. Mullen, and L. W. Green. 1992. A meta-analysis of studies of the health belief model with adults. *Health Education Research* 7(1):107-116.

Hassenteufel, P. 2008. *Sociologie politique: L'action publique.* Paris: Armand Colin.

Hawe, P., A. Shiell, and T. Riley. 2004. Complex interventions: How "out of control" can a randomised controlled trial be? *BMJ* 328(7455):1561-1563.

HHS (U.S. Department of Health and Human Services). No date. *Planned approach to community health: Guide for the local coordinator.* http://www.lgreen.net/patch.pdf (accessed June 4, 2012).

Hochbaum, G. M. 1956. Why people seek diagnostic X-rays. *Public Health Reports* 71(4):377-380.

Hochbaum, G. M. 1959. *Public participation in medical screening program.* Washington, DC: U.S. Department of Health, Education, and Welfare, Public Health Service.

Hopkins, D. 2001. Recommendations regarding interventions to reduce tobacco use and exposure to environmental tobacco smoke. *American Journal of Preventive Medicine* 20(2):10-15.

Hopkins, D. P., P. A. Briss, C. J. Ricard, C. G. Husten, V. G. Carande-Kulis, J. E. Fielding, M. O. Alao, J. W. McKenna, D. J. Sharp, and J. R. Harris. 2001. Reviews of evidence regarding interventions to reduce tobacco use and exposure to environmental tobacco smoke. *American Journal of Preventive Medicine* 20(2):16-66.

Howlett, M., M. Ramesh, and A. Perl. 2009. *Studying public policy: Policy cycles and policy subsystems*. Don Mills, Ontario: Oxford University Press.

Inayatullah, S. 2011. City futures in transformation: Emerging issues and case studies. *Futures* 43(7):654-661.

IOM (Institute of Medicine). 1999. *Gulf War veterans: Measuring health*. Washington, DC: National Academy Press.

IOM. 2000a. *Clearing the air: Asthma and indoor air exposures*. Washington, DC: National Academy Press.

IOM. 2000b. *Promoting health: Intervention strategies from social and behavioral research*. Washington, DC: National Academy Press.

IOM. 2002. *The future of the public's health in the 21st century*. Washington, DC: The National Academies Press.

IOM. 2003. *Who will keep the public healthy?: Educating public health professionals for the 21st century*. Washington, DC: The National Academies Press.

IOM. 2011. *For the public's health: Revitalizing law and policy to meet new challenges*. Washington, DC: The National Academies Press.

Israel, B. A., B. Checkoway, A. Schulz, and M. Zimmerman. 1994. Health education and community empowerment: Conceptualizing and measuring perceptions of individual, organizational, and community control. *Health Education and Behavior* 21(2):149-170.

Janz, N. K., and M. H. Becker. 1984. The Health Belief Model: A decade later. *Health Education and Behavior* 11(1):1-47.

Kawachi, I., and L. Berkman. 2001. Social ties and mental health. *Journal of Urban Health* 78(3):458-467.

Kawachi, I., and L. Berkman. 2003. *Neighborhoods and health*. New York: Oxford University Press.

Kickbusch, I. 2003. The contribution of the World Health Organization to a new public health and health promotion. *American Journal of Public Health* 93(3):383-388.

Kickbusch, I., and L. Payne. 2003. Twenty-first century health promotion: The public health revolution meets the wellness revolution. *Health Promotion International* 18(4):275-278.

Kindig, D., and G. Stoddart. 2003. What is population health? *American Journal of Public Health* 93(3):380-383.

Kreisel, W., and Y. V. Schirnding. 1998. Intersectoral action for health: A cornerstone for health for all in the 21st century. *World Health Statistics Quarterly* 51(1):75-75.

Kreuter, M. W. 1992. PATCH: Its origin, basic concepts, and links to contemporary public health policy. *Journal of Health Education* 23(3):135-139.

Kreuter, M. W., N. A. Lezin, M. W. Kreuter, and L. W. Green. 1997. *Community health promotion ideas that work: A field-book for practitioners*. Boston: Jones and Bartlett Publishers.

Kreuter, M. W., N. A. Lezin, and L. A. Young. 2000. Evaluating community-based collaborative mechanisms: Implications for practitioners. *Health Promotion Practice* 1(1):49-63.

Larsen, E. L., and L. Manderson. 2009. "A good spot": Health promotion discourse, healthy cities and heterogeneity in contemporary Denmark. *Health and Place* 15(2):606-613.

Lefebvre, R. C., and J. A. Flora. 1988. Social marketing and public health intervention *Health Education Quarterly* 15(3):299-315.

Lionberger, H. F. 1964. *Application of diffusion research in agriculture to heart disease control.* Berkeley, CA: California State Department of Public Health.

Livingood, W. C., J. P. Allegrante, C. O. Airhihenbuwa, N. M. Clark, R. C. Windsor, M. A. Zimmerman, and L. W. Green. 2011. Applied social and behavioral science to address complex health problems. *American Journal of Preventive Medicine* 41(5):525-531.

Mabry, P. L., D. H. Olster, G. D. Morgan, and D. B. Abrams. 2008. Interdisciplinarity and systems science to improve population health: A view from the NIH Office of Behavioral and Social Sciences Research. *American Journal of Preventive Medicine* 35(2 Suppl):S211-S224.

Marmot, M. G., and R. Wilkerson. 2000. *Social determinants of health.* New York: Oxford University Press.

McGinnis, J. M., and W. H. Foege. 1993. Actual causes of death in the United States. *JAMA* 270(18):2207-2212.

McIntyre, S., and A. Ellaway. 2000. Ecological approaches: Rediscovering the role of the physical and social environment. In *Social epidemiology*, edited by L. Berkman and I. Kawachi. New York: Oxford University Press. Pp. 332-348.

McLaren, L., and P. Hawe. 2005. Ecological perspectives in health research. *Journal of Epidemiology and Community Health* 59(1):6-14.

McLaren, L., L. M. Ghali, D. Lorenzetti, and M. Rock. 2007. Out of context? Translating evidence from the North Karelia Project over place and time. *Health Education Research* 22(3):414-424.

McLeroy, K. R., D. Bibeau, A. Steckler, and K. Glanz. 1988. An ecological perspective on health promotion programs. *Health Education and Behavior* 15(4):351-377.

Mercer, S. L., B. J. DeVinney, L. J. Fine, L. W. Green, and D. Dougherty. 2007. Study designs for effectiveness and translation research: Identifying trade-offs. *American Journal of Preventive Medicine* 33(2):139-154.

Mokdad, A. H., J. S. Marks, D. F. Stroup, and J. L. Gerberding. 2004. Actual causes of death in the United States, 2000. *JAMA* 291(10):1238-1245.

Mokdad, A. H., J. S. Marks, D. F. Stroup, and J. L. Gerberding. 2005. Correction: Actual causes of death in the United States, 2000. *JAMA: The Journal of the American Medical Association* 293(3):293-294.

Moynihan, D. P. 1969. *Maximum feasible misunderstanding: Community action in the war on poverty.* New York: Macmillan.

NCI (National Cancer Institute). 2000. *State and local legislative action to reduce tobacco use.* Bethesda, MD: National Institutes of Health.

Nelson, M. C., P. Gordon-Larsen, Y. Song, and B. M. Popkin. 2006. Built and social environments: Associations with adolescent overweight and activity. *American Journal of Preventive Medicine* 31(2):109-117.

Norris, S. L., P. J. Nichols, C. J. Caspersen, R. E. Glasgow, M. M. Engelgau, L. Jack, S. R. Snyder, V. G. Carande-Kulis, G. Isham, and S. Garfield. 2002. Increasing diabetes self-management education in community settings: A systematic review. *American Journal of Preventive Medicine* 22(4):39-66.

Nurmagambetov, T. A., S. B. L. Barnett, V. Jacob, S. K. Chattopadhyay, D. P. Hopkins, D. D. Crocker, G. G. Dumitru, and S. Kinyota. 2011. Economic value of home-based, multi-trigger, multicomponent interventions with an environmental focus for reducing asthma morbidity: A community guide systematic review. *American Journal of Preventive Medicine* 41(2):S33-S47.

Nutbeam, D. 1998a. Evaluating health promotion—progress, problems and solutions. *Health Promotion International* 13(1):27-44.

Nutbeam, D. 1998b. Health promotion glossary. *Health Promotion International* 13(4):349-364.

Nutbeam, D. 2000. Health literacy as a public health goal: A challenge for contemporary health education and communication strategies into the 21st century. *Health Promotion International* 15(3):259-267.

Office on Smoking and Health. 1999. *Best practices for comprehensive tobacco control programs.* Atlanta, GA: Centers for Disease Control and Prevention.

Office on Smoking and Health. 2007. *Best practices for comprehensive tobacco control programs.* Atlanta, GA: Centers for Disease Control and Prevention.

Ottoson, J. M., L. W. Green, W. L. Beery, S. K. Senter, C. L. Cahill, D. C. Pearson, H. P. Greenwald, R. Hamre, and L. Leviton. 2009. Policy-contribution assessment and field-building analysis of the Robert Wood Johnson Foundation's active living research program. *American Journal of Preventive Medicine* 36(2):S34-S43.

Owen, R., D. Kendrick, C. Mulvaney, T. Coleman, and S. Royal. 2011. Non-legislative interventions for the promotion of cycle helmet wearing by children. *Cochrane Library* 2:CD003985.

Patrick, D. L., and T. M. Wickizer. 1995. Community and health. In *Society and health*, edited by B. Amick III, S. Levine, A. R. Tarlov, and D. Chapman-Walsh. New York: Oxford University Press.

Pierce, J. P., and E. A. Gilpin. 2004. How did the Master Settlement Agreement change tobacco industry expenditures for cigarette advertising and promotions? *Health Promotion Practice* 5(3 Suppl):84S-90S.

Poland, J. C., L. W. Green, and I. Rootman. 2000. *Settings in health promotion: Linking theory and practice.* Thousand Oaks, CA: Sage.

Potvin, L., and C. M. Jones. 2011. Twenty-five years after the Ottawa Charter: The critical role of health promotion for public health. *Canadian Journal of Public Health* 102(4):244-248.

Potvin, L., and L. Richard. 2001. The evaluation of community health promotion programmes. In *Evaluation in health promotion: Principles and perspectives*, edited by I. Rootman, M. Goodstadt, D. V. Hyndman, L. McQueen, L. Potvin, J. Springett and E. Ziglio. Copenhagen: WHO Regional Publications. Pp. 213-240.

Puska, P., and A. Uutela. 2000. Community intervention in cardiovascular health promotion: North Karelia, 1972-1999. In *Integrating behavioral and social sciences with public health*, edited by N. Schneiderman, M. A. Speers, J. M. Silva, H. Tomes, and J. H. Gentry. Baltimore, MD: United Book Press, Inc. Pp. 73-96.

Puska, P., A. Nissinen, J. Tuomilehto, J. T. Salonen, K. Koskela, A. McAlister, T. E. Kottke, N. Maccoby, and J. W. Farquhar. 1985. The community-based strategy to prevent coronary heart disease: Conclusions from the ten years of the North Karelia Project. *Annual Review of Public Health* 6(1):147-193.

Puska, P., E. Vartiainen, J. Tuomilehto, V. Salomaa, and A. Nissinen. 1998. Changes in premature deaths in Finland: Successful long-term prevention of cardiovascular diseases. *Bulletin of the World Health Organization* 76(4):419-425.

Puska, P., E. Vartiainen, T. Laatikainen, P. Jousilahti, and M. Paavola. 2009. *The North Karelia Project: From North Karelia to national action.* Helsinki: Helsinki University Printing House.

Reininger, B., D. W. Martin, M. Ross, S. Pamela Smith, and T. Dinh-Zarr. 2005. Advancing the theory and measurement of collective empowerment: A qualitative study. *International Quarterly of Community Health Education* 25(3):211-238.

Reynolds, L. 2012. "No decision about me, without me": A place for social marketing within the new public health architecture? *Perspectives in Public Health* 132(1):26-30.

Richard, L., L. Potvin, N. Kishchuk, H. Prlic, and L. W. Green. 1996. Assessment of the integration of the ecological approach in health promotion programs. *American Journal of Health Promotion* 10(4):318-328.

Richard, L., L. Gauvin, and K. Raine. 2011. Ecological models revisited: Their uses and evolution in health promotion over two decades. *Annual Review of Public Health* 32:307-326.

Ritchie, L. D., S. Sharma, J. P. Ikeda, R. A. Mitchell, A. Raman, B. S. Green, M. L. Hudes, and S. E. Fleming. 2010. Study protocol taking action together: A YMCA-based protocol to prevent type-2 diabetes in high-BMI inner-city African-American children. *Trials* 11:60.

Rogers, E. M. 2002. The nature of technology transfer. *Science Communication* 23(3):323-341.

Rootman, I., M. Goodstadt, L. Potvin, and J. Springett. 2001. A framework for health promotion evaluation. In *Evluation in health promotoin: Principles and Perspectives*, edited by I. Rootman, M. Goodstadt, B. Hyndman, D. V. McQueen, L. Potvin, J. Springett, and E. Ziglio. Copenhagen, Denmark: WHO. Pp. 7-43.

Rose, G. 1992. *A strategy of preventive medicine.* Oxford: Oxford University Press.

Rossi, A. S. 2001. *Caring and doing for others: Social responsibility in the domains of family, work, and community.* Chicago, IL: University of Chicago Press.

Rothman, J., and E. R. Brown. 1989. Indicators of societal action to promote social health. In *Health promotion indicators and actions*, edited by S. B. Kar. New York: Springer.

Sallis, S. E., N. Owen, and E. B. Fisher Jr. 2008. Echological models of health behavior. In *Health behavior and health education: Theory, research, and practice*, 4th ed., edited by K. Glantz, B. K. Rimer, and K. Viswanath. San Francisco, CA: JosseyBass. Pp. 465-486.

Samuels, S. E. 1993. Project LEAN—lessons learned from a national social marketing campaign. *Public Health Reports* 108(1):45-53.

Simons-Morton, B. G., G. S. Parcel, and N. M. O'Hara. 1988a. Implementing organizational changes to promote healthful diet and physical activity at school. *Health Education and Behavior* 15(1):115-130.

Simons-Morton, B. G., G. S. Parcel, and N. M. O'Hara. 1988b. *Promoting physical activity among adults: A CDC community intervention handbook.* Atlanta, GA: Centers for Disease Control and Prevention, National Center for Chronic Disease Prevention and Health Promotion.

Simons-Morton, D. G., B. G. Simons-Morton, G. S. Parcel, and J. F. Bunker. 1988c. Influencing personal and environmental conditions for community health: A multilevel intervention model. *Family and Community Health* 11(2):25-35.

Simons-Morton, B. G., S. G. Brink, D. G. Simons-Morton, R. M. McIntyre, M. Chapman, J. Longoria, and G. S. Parcel. 1989. An ecological approach to the prevention of injuries due to drinking and driving. *Health Education and Behavior* 16(3):397-411.

Simons-Morton, B. G., S. G. Brink, G. S. Parcel, and D. G. Simons-Morton. 1991. *Preventing alcohol-related health problems among adolescents and young adults: A CDC intervention handbook.* Atlanta, GA: Centers for Disease Control and Prevention.

Simons-Morton, B. G., W. H. Greene, and N. H. Gottlieb. 1995. *Introduction to health education and health promotion.* Prospect Heights, IL: Waveland Press.

Smith, W. A. 2000. Social marketing: An evolving definition. *American Journal of Health Behavior* 24(1):11-17.

Spencer, B., U. Broesskamp-Stone, B. Ruckstuhl, G. Ackermann, A. Spoerri, and B. Cloetta. 2008. Modelling the results of health promotion activities in Switzerland: Development of the Swiss Model for outcome classification in health promotion and prevention. *Health Promotion International* 23(1):86-97.

Spinks, A., C. Turner, J. Nixon, and R. J. McClure. 2009. The WHO Safe Communities Model for the prevention of injury in whole populations. *Cochrane Database of Systematic Reviews* 3: CD004445.

Stansfeld, S., J. Head, and J. Ferrie. 1999. Short-term disability, sickness absence, and social gradients in the Whitehall II study. *International Journal of Law and Psychiatry* 22(5-6):425-439.

Stokols, D. 1992. Establishing and maintaining healthy environments. Toward a social ecology of health promotion. *American Psychologist* 47(1):6-22.

Stokols, D. 1996. Translating social ecological theory into guidelines for community health promotion. *American Journal of Health Promotion* 10(4):282-298.

Stokols, D., J. Allen, and R. L. Bellingham. 1996. The social ecology of health promotion: Implications for research and practice. *American Journal of Health Promotion* 10(4):247-251.

Suser, M. 1995. The tribulations of trials—Interventions in communities. *American Journal of Public Health* 85:156-158.

Syme, S. L. 1994. The social environment and health. *Daedalus* 123(4):79-86.

Task Force on Community Preventive Services. 2005. Tobacco. In *The guide to community preventive services: What works to promote health?*, edited by S. Zaza, P. A. Briss, and K. W. Harris. New York: Oxford University Press. Pp. 3-79.

Thorpe, K. E., and Z. Yang. 2011. Enrolling people with prediabetes ages 60-64 in a proven weight loss program could save Medicare $7 billion or more. *Health Affairs* 30(9):1673-1679.

Tirodkar, M. A., D. W. Baker, N. Khurana, G. Makoul, M. W. Paracha, and N. R. Kandula. 2010. Explanatory models of coronary heart disease among South Asian immigrants. *Patient Education and Counseling* 85(2):230-236.

Tobacco Education and Research Oversight Committee. 2009. *Endangered investment: Toward a tobacco-free California, 2009-2011*. Sacramento, CA: Tobacco Education and Research Oversight Committee.

Traynor, M. P., M. E. Begay, and S. A. Glantz. 1993. New tobacco industry strategy to prevent local tobacco control. *JAMA* 270(4):479-486.

Vasudevan, V., S. S. Nambisan, A. K. Singh, and T. Pearl. 2009. Effectiveness of media and enforcement campaigns in increasing seat belt usage rates in a state with a secondary seat belt law. *Traffic Injury Prevention* 10(4):330-339.

Wagner, E. H., T. M. Wickizer, A. Cheadle, B. M. Psaty, T. D. Koepsell, P. Diehr, S. J. Curry, M. Von Korff, C. Anderman, and W. L. Beery. 2000. The Kaiser Family Foundation Community Health Promotion Grants Program: Findings from an outcome evaluation. *Health Services Research* 35(3):561-589.

WHO (World Health Organization). 1986. *The Ottawa Charter for health promotion*. Geneva: World Health Organization.

WHO. 2010. *The Adelaide Statement on Health in All Policy: Moving towards a shared governance for health and well being*. Geneva: World Health Organization.

Winkleby, M. A. 1994. The future of community-based cardiovascular disease intervention studies. *American Journal of Public Health* 84(9):1369-1372.

Winkleby, M. A., C. B. Taylor, D. Jatulis, and S. P. Fortmann. 1996. The long-term effects of a cardiovascular disease prevention trial: The Stanford Five-City Project. *American Journal of Public Health* 86(12):1773-1779.

Worthman, C. M. 1999. Epidemiology of human development. In *Hormones, health, and behaviors: A socio-ecological and lifespan perspective*, edited by C. Panter-Brick and C. M. Worthman. Cambridge: Cambridge University Press. Pp. 47-104.

3

Community-Based Prevention:
More Than the Sum of Its Parts

This chapter discusses how the methods of systems science can help increase understanding about the complexity of community-based prevention intervention by disentangling important features and associated variables, clarifying whether and how each of the variables changes over time, identifying causal relationships among the variables, quantifying the variables and the causal relationships, and simulating how changes to the system affect the variables and causal relationships in the system. Domains of value (health, community well-being, and community process) and illustrative elements within each domain are discussed, as are issues in valuing resources and costs of community-based prevention.

As discussed in Chapter 2, community-based prevention interventions cover a broad spectrum of types, from those directed at a specific health condition (e.g., high blood pressure or diabetes) to those aimed at a much broader and more complex array of conditions, including the prevalence of chronic and infectious diseases; the social, economic, and environmental determinants of population health; and health disparities and inequities experienced by lower income, lower educational status, and racial and ethnic minority populations. Chapter 2 also discussed the ecological model and pointed out the existence of multiple determinants of health at multiple levels that interact and link with each other. However, prevailing approaches to funding, research, and practice associated with community-based prevention interventions often fail to recognize their inherent complexity. For instance, categorical funding programs promote a one-disease-at-a-time vision (with an accompanying set of interventions) for improving population health behaviors and health outcomes. Similarly, many research and evaluation questions seek to identify the best intervention or to examine interventions in the context of a single behavioral or health outcome. And, in the field, approaches to policy and practice change often reflect the interests of the institutions or organizations leading the efforts (e.g., government agencies, community-based organizations, or advocacy groups).

Current approaches tend to focus on individual rather than comprehensive interventions, to attribute changes in health behaviors and health outcomes to specific interventions instead of multiple or synergistic efforts, to not assess effectiveness and costs in terms of the collective value of multi-component intervention approaches, and to guide decisions about priorities and allocate resources intervention by intervention in line with these types of evidence. As such, prevailing approaches fall short in depicting the collective impact of community-based prevention efforts (Hanleybrown et al., 2012; Kania and Kramer, 2011).

However, there has been a growing amount of attention paid to new approaches to address these dynamic and complex systems (Homer and Hirsch, 2006; Luke and Stamatakis, 2012; Mabry et al., 2008; Madon et al., 2007). Examples include the community transformation grants from the Centers for Disease Control and Prevention (CDC); intervention and applied research efforts such as community-based participatory research; the dissemination and implementation research supported by the NIH National Heart, Lung, and Blood Institute and the Office of Behavioral and Social Sciences Research; and cross-sector and multidisciplinary interventions, such as the CDC Communities Putting Prevention to Work program and the Healthy Kids Healthy Communities program (BSSR/NIH, 2012; CDC, 2012a,b; Horowitz et al., 2009; NHLBI/NIH, 2012; RWJF, 2012).

Systems science methods have the potential for overcoming some of the problems with current approaches. Systems science is the study of "dynamic interrelationships of variables at multiple levels of analysis (e.g., from cells to society) simultaneously (often through causal feedback processes), while also studying the impact on the behavior of the system as a whole over time."[1] For purposes of this report, a *system* will refer to the interrelationships of relevant elements, resources, and processes that characterize community-based prevention. Systems science approaches excel at identifying nonlinear relationships, bidirectional feedback loops, time-delayed effects, emergent properties of systems, and oscillating system behavior (Mabry et al., 2010).

---

[1] As defined by the Office of Behavioral and Social Sciences Research at the National Institutes of Health: http://obssr.od.nih.gov/scientific_areas/methodology/systems_science/index.aspx (accessed July 5, 2012).

Systems thinking is increasingly associated with community-based prevention, notably in obesity control. Of major importance from a systems science perspective is the context in which those interventions take place, that is, the social systems that are imbedded in and interacting with other social systems. Second, there is a growing literature that uses the system metaphor to describe the structure and functioning of the intervention itself (IOM, 2010; Livingood et al., 2011; Trickett, 2009). Because of the complexity, comprehensiveness, and intersectoral, and context-responsive nature of the broader community-based prevention efforts, a systems perspective is well equipped to provide needed analytical descriptions and evaluations of the multiple transformations targeted by such programs, policies, and strategies.

Using a systems science approach to think about community-based prevention can help people think through all the links that may be involved in and affected by a change in the community, whether that change comes from a deliberate intervention or a trend, (such as more smoking or less exercise) caused by forces that may lie outside the community. Furthermore, systems science can help further elucidate

- the pathways through which policy, system, and environmental changes operate to affect population health.
- important ingredients that are needed to implement effective community-based prevention interventions as well as the implementation fidelity and "dose" of these activities (Carroll et al., 2007; Glasgow et al., 1999; Linnan and Steckler, 2002).
- methods needed to capture multi-component and dynamic community trends and to triangulate different qualitative and quantitative data sources (Patton, 2002; Rossi et al., 2004; Teddlie and Tashakkori, 2009; Ulin et al., 2005).
- the extent to which scale-up and spread of evidence-based interventions may be limited by the need to customize these strategies to local political or environmental circumstances, resource constraints, populations (e.g., race and ethnicity, poverty, urban versus rural, youth versus adult), and settings (e.g., home, child care, school, work, community).
- the challenges posed by political, social, and economic forces to the structures (e.g., partners, resources) and processes (e.g., participation, decision making) associated with collaborative community approaches to planning, implementing, enforcing, evaluating, and sustaining these prevention interventions.

Systems science methods are designed to deal with complexity and could prove particularly useful in analyzing community-based prevention interventions and their impacts (Hammond, 2009; Huang et al., 2009). Results of the application of systems science methods could prove useful in valuing community-based prevention because they can provide information about not only the intervention programs, policies, and associated outcomes but also the contextual conditions, the multi-cause nature of change, and the dynamic interactions among all of the factors.

APPLYING SYSTEMS SCIENCE TO COMMUNITY-BASED PREVENTION

Systems science methods can be used to explore the various pathways leading from community-based prevention interventions to improvements in population behavioral and health outcomes, such as the influence of a sugar-sweetened beverage tax on the purchase and consumption of foods and beverages. Such methods can also capture the variation in these pathways associated with contextual factors (such as population characteristics, concentration of fast food restaurants, employment opportunities, and living wages) and detect changes in the overall system as new interventions surface.

Systems science methods can address both detail and dynamic complexity. With respect to detail complexity, these methods can clarify assumptions about public health problems, local community context, and change strategies and processes by identifying the variables and the underlying causal relationships among the variables. At the same time these methods are designed to examine how causal structures change over time, including the effect of changes in the type or number of interventions implemented, changes in social norms and community practices, changes in leadership or staff, and so on. Examining these causal structures can help identify the system leverage points that have the greatest potential for affecting behavioral and health outcomes, can increase understanding about intended effects and unintended consequences of the interventions implemented, and can identify facilitating factors and challenges influencing community change processes (Meadows, 1999; Sterman, 2000; Ulrich, 2000).

For examples of systems science approaches to valuing community-based prevention interventions, see Appendix B.

VALUING COMMUNITY-BASED PREVENTION: DOMAINS AND ELEMENTS

Policy makers, funders, and relevant stakeholders make decisions about the value of community-based interventions. Traditional approaches to assess value tend to focus solely on health impacts, to value interventions in isolation, to overlook community processes, and to fail to monitor pathways toward progress. The committee was asked to develop a framework for assessing the value of community-based prevention. Because of the way in which community-based prevention is designed and developed (e.g., often to address the social and environmental determinants of health), the committee concluded that impacts of these interventions go beyond health effects. Therefore, a framework for valuing community-based prevention needs to take into account not only the outcomes in the domain of health, but also the outcomes in areas other than health. A framework that does not take into account and value non-health outcomes would be counting all the costs but not all the benefits, thereby providing an inaccurate and inadequate picture of the value of community-based prevention. To assess the true value of community-based prevention, therefore, decision makers, funders, and stakeholders would benefit from an approach that looks not just at health impacts, but at other impacts as well.

A major task facing the committee, then, was determining what domains should be included in a framework to value community-based prevention interventions. As a first step, each committee member was asked to list the outcomes he or she thought could result from community-based prevention interventions. The list generated included more than 100 items and all acknowledged that not everything that could be valued appeared on the list. As a next step, the committee decided to group the items into major categories. Clearly, a major outcome of community-based prevention is its impact on health. Therefore, health was identified as a major domain of interest.

However, there were a number of other items on the list that did not fall neatly into a health domain, for example, education, income, green space, crime, social support, and workplace safety. Initially, the committee identified six major categories under which these other items could be grouped: social environment, physical environment, economics, equity, employment, and education. Yet, as the committee discussed these items and reviewed the literature, it became clear that these elements were all elements related to well-being. Therefore, the committee identified a second major domain as the domain of community well-being.

There were a number of items that did not fit readily into either the health category or the well-being category but which the committee identified as important items of value, including such things as leadership, skill building, and civic participation. An examination of the history of community health efforts demonstrates that various process elements (such as skill building, leadership, and participation) are features that account for the relative success of community-based programs. Early efforts in the first half of the 20th century involved engaging stakeholder organizations and affected populations in first, the support of planned programs, then in actually planning programs, then in evaluating programs, and finally in community-based participatory research (CBPR) (Green, 1986).

Based on the literature of CBPR (e.g., Minkler and Wallerstein, 2008) the committee deliberately decided to identify community process as a specific area of valued outcomes for community-based prevention.

Elements in the community process domain inherently affect outcomes upstream (e.g., civic participation) that, in turn, affect outcomes downstream (e.g., policy adoption and implementation), further downstream (e.g., equitable access to environments or resources to support health), further downstream (e.g., healthy behaviors of citizens in these environments or use of these resources), further downstream (e.g., healthy lifestyle choices of citizens), and, ultimately, health (although health feeds back to greater capacity for civic participation). Therefore, the committee concludes community process should be identified as a separate domain because in many cases, community empowerment and community capacity have been shown to be valued by communities in their own right (Sandoval et al., 2011). Also, because process elements are intermediary outcomes that increase well-being and health interventions (Minkler et al., 2008; Viswanathan et al., 2004), failing to recognize the increase of such potential as a valued outcome will further disadvantage those communities whose structural and population characteristics put them at increased risk of health and well-being deficit. It is important to note that without a solid grounding in science, community process, as is the case with any democratic process, could lead to worse outcomes with respect to health and well-being.

This section of Chapter 3 describes in more detail the wide array of effects that community-based prevention can have, grouping them under the three distinct but interrelated categories of outcomes, or *domains of value*: health, community well-being, and community process. The committee is aware that health is a component of well-being but for purposes of this report the health component is separated from other elements of community well-being because health is a particular outcome of interest. The goal in valuing these domains is to account for all of the potential harms and benefits of community-based interventions as well as the possible savings and costs associated with the interventions. This section introduces the domains of value as well as associated elements.

It is important to note that the list of elements included in each domain below is meant to be illustrative. The actual elements selected for valuing will depend on the particular intervention and its implementation. It is unlikely that any given intervention will have value in all elements listed, and there may well be other elements not listed here that should be included. The committee has identified one element, equity, that crosses all domains.

Health

Physical health includes mortality, morbidity, and functional capability. Mental health includes cognition, individual resilience or emotional reserves, mortality due to such causes as suicide, morbidity (e.g., depression), and socio-emotional health-related quality of life (e.g., stress, behaviors, injuries, and perceptions of health). The promotion of mental and physical health includes several elements, in particular, reductions in the incidence and prevalence of disease, declines in mortality, and increases in health-related quality of life. Equity is another important element in the health domain. It is well documented that significant health disparities exist by race, ethnicity, and socioeconomic status (SES) (AHRQ, 2012; APHA, no date; IOM, 2003). Health inequalities across demographic groups (e.g., by race, ethnicity, gender, and SES) may be caused by inequalities in access to health care, by the unequal effect of public measures aimed at risk reduction, or by the unequal distribution of various social determinants of health (e.g., education, income and wealth, opportunity and liberty) (AHRQ, 2012; IOM, 2003, 2009). It may be, however, that the two goals of health policy—improving population health in the aggregate and distributing health fairly—are in tension. For example, some efforts that improve population health in the aggregate may increase health inequalities between groups, for example, a campaign to improve prenatal care that primarily reaches middle to higher income women and is not effective among lower income women may well increase health disparities. Reasonable people may disagree about when to give priority to one goal over the other. However, when assessing value, health inequalities are one element to consider.

The charge to the committee specified a focus on the prevention of long-term chronic diseases. As noted throughout the report, long-term chronic illnesses are often the result of a complex, extended interaction between genetics, individual behaviors, and environments. This complexity can make the task of valuing more difficult. For example, behaviors, such as eating foods with minimal nutritional value and participating in sedentary activities that can lead to obesity and related chronic diseases, are generally the result of lifestyles shaped in part by an individual's environment. Lifestyle interventions aimed at preventing certain diseases, such as cardiovascular disease (CVD) and diabetes, have been shown to be effective (Saha et al., 2010). However, lowering the prevalence of CVD and diabetes is an outcome that takes a long time to realize. Interventions aimed at such outcomes can produce intermediate markers, such as decreased insulin resistance or lower blood pressure. For long-term outcomes such as the prevention of chronic disease, it will be important to identify intermediate or proximal outcomes as part of the valuation and determination of progress.

Community Well-Being

Community well-being is a valued outcome in and of itself. Independent of the health of individuals in a community, the concept of community well-being has been used to account for elements associated with community context, or the social, economic, and physical environments characterizing the community (IOM, 2009). Elements of community well-being include wealth and income, education, employment, safety, transportation, housing, worksites, food, health care, and recreational spaces, among others. These elements are produced, reproduced, and transformed by the practice of individuals in the community. Their benefits accrue to both individuals and the community as a whole.

Physical Environment

Frumkin (2003) writes of the "*atmosphere* of a place, the quality of its *environment*" and the effect that it can have on both health and well-being. He identified four aspects of the built environment that may have an impact on human health and community well-being: nature contact, buildings, public spaces, and urban form. The built environment includes how land is used, the quality of housing and other buildings, transportation, and other design features "that together provide opportunities for travel and physical activity" and, more broadly, an environment that "is designed and constructed by humans" (IOM, 2001; TRB/IOM, 2005).

Land use, urban form, and green space The composition of the built environment, Frumkin's "urban form," has been associated with a number of health effects. For example, physical characteristics of neighborhoods have been found to be associated with lower levels of physical exercise and an increased risk of obesity (Ewing et al., 2006; Lopez, 2004; Nelson et al., 2006). The presence or absence of amenities, particularly the opportunities to buy healthy affordable food, can also have an effect on health (Bodor et al., 2010; Leung et al., 2011; Michimi and Wimberly, 2010; Morland et al., 2006; Powell et al., 2007). Access to—or even the presence of—green space is associated with increased physical activity, better perceived general health, mitigation of the effects of stressful life events, and lower prevalence of some illnesses (Ellaway, 2005; Maas et al., 2006, 2009; Ulrich, 1984; Van Den Berg et al., 2010).

Urban form also has effects beyond those on health. For example, areas with a high degree of "walkability" are perceived to be more aesthetically pleasing and are associated with more unplanned interactions with others and a greater sense of community (Wood et al., 2010). Trees in cities allow for greater energy conservation and lower heating and cooling costs for buildings (McPherson et al., 1997).

Transportation Numerous studies have found that using public transit increases physical activity (Besser and Dannenberg, 2005; Lachapelle and Frank, 2009; Weinstein and Schimek, 2005; Wener and Evans, 2007). MacDonald and colleagues (2010) found that commuting to work by light rail was associated with a reduction in body mass index and reduced odds of becoming obese. Active travel, such as walking and cycling, along with increasing physical activity can also lead to a decrease in vehicle emissions, thereby improving air quality (de Nazelle, 2011). Investment in public transportation has other benefits as well—for example, bringing jobs and economic activity to communities (Weisbrod and Reno, 2009).

Building quality (indoor air) Housing is another area that has effects on both health and community well-being. People spend most of their time indoors, making buildings a component of the built environment that can have a significant impact on an individual's health. Indoor air can contain radon, environmental tobacco smoke, and thousands of other chemicals and biological contaminants that pose serious risks to health (EPA, 2001). Children, in particular, are at risk of harm from indoor and outdoor air pollution, and the impact can be lifelong (Barakat-Haddad et al., 2012; EPA, 2001). A 2011 IOM committee found that "poor indoor environmental quality is creating health problems today and impairs the ability of occupants to work and learn" (IOM, 2011a, p. 7). In addition to its health benefits, providing quality housing also brings benefits to the community in the form of such things as improved educational outcomes and reduced crime (Carlson et al., 2011).

Social and Economic Environments

Education Extensive research has demonstrated the link between education and health outcomes throughout the life course (IOM, 2006a; Lleras-Muney, 2005). Researchers have also documented the relationship of education and well-being (i.e., higher earnings, higher percentages of home ownership and second-car ownership, reduced crime, reduced welfare, reduced unemployment and reduced poverty (Barnett, 1985, 1996; Gorey, 2001; Schweinhart et al., 1993).

Employment/unemployment Unemployment is positively associated with mortality from all causes, with both physical and mental illness, and with the increased use of health care services (Haan and Myck, 2009; Jin et al.,

1995; Rueda et al., 2012; Strully, 2009; Wilkinson and Marmot, 2003). Employment also has numerous non-health effects. For example, it is associated with more marriage, less divorce, more marital happiness, and greater child well-being (White and Rogers, 2000). Decreases in the unemployment rate have been found to be associated with declines in property crime rates (Raphael and Winter-Ebmer, 2001). Rising unemployment increases the incidence of foster home placement (Catalano et al., 1999).

Crime/safety Research has associated increased physical activity with increased feelings of neighborhood safety (Harrison et al., 2007). Conversely, those living in high crime areas were more likely to smoke and to report poorer health, poor sleep habits, and less exercise (Johnson et al., 2009; Shareck and Ellaway, 2011). In terms of non-health effects, crime and the fear of violence can interfere with social interaction and trust among community members. For example, crime or the fear of crime has been found to limit women's movement around their environment and to increase levels of mistrust and fear, (Keane, 1998; Ross and Jang, 2000). Milam and colleagues (2010) found that math and reading achievement in schools decreased significantly with increasing neighborhood violence.

Social support and social networks Social networks are defined as webs of person-centered ties (Berkman and Glass, 2000). Numerous research studies have shown the relationship of social support and social networks to both physical and mental health (Berkman and Glass, 2000; Berkman and Kawachi, 2000; Cohen et al., 2000; Cornwell and Waite, 2009; Kawachi and Berkman, 2003; Marmot and Wilkinson, 1999; Maulik et al., 2009; Stansfeld et al., 1999). However, in addition to their relationship to health, social networks and social support are important in and of themselves. For example, Skogan (1989) found that neighborhoods in which residents have organizations and social support resources upon which to draw have more opportunity for action in "defense of their community." Research has also shown that positive academic outcomes are promoted by social support (Garnefski and Diekstra, 1996; Malecki and Demaray, 2007).

Social cohesion Social cohesion has been characterized by Marmot and Wilkinson (1999) as including "mutual trust and respect between different sections of society." Social cohesion has been shown to be positively associated with health and levels of physical activity (Cradock et al., 2009; Kim et al., 2008; Lindén-Boström et al., 2010; Marmot and Wilkinson, 1999). But social cohesion also has important effects beyond those on health. For example, areas with higher levels of social cohesion are associated with lower levels of crime, with increasing contributions to group goals, and with economic prosperity (Hirschfield and Bowers, 1997; Shimizu, 2011; Stanley, 2003).

Equity As mentioned previously, equity is an important element that crosses all three domains. Elements of community well-being are often not equitably distributed in a community. For example, both education and wealth, which are elements of the social environment, are often distributed unequally by race, and considerable attention has been given in recent literature to growing inequalities in income and wealth. The same point may be made for social trust: Levels may vary across various groups in a society, and some practices may weaken trust across groups. The built environment in a society may also be inequitable in its impact on different groups—neighborhoods may vary in the quality of housing, green space, transportation, or even access to fresh food. It is important in valuing community well-being to focus not only on aggregate measures, but also on how community well-being is distributed. Inequity in the distribution of these aspects of community well-being may lead to inequities in the distribution of health and may also contribute to inequities in community processes.

Community Processes

Community-based prevention involves decisions among groups of people about how to live in society, how cities are built, what food is served in schools, and so on. Therefore, it is important that the process by which an intervention is adopted and undertaken be treated as a valued outcome. With a vaccination, effectiveness does not depend on whether the patient trusts the doctor. In contrast, the success of a healthful eating campaign may hinge on the level of trust in the process.

Community processes refer to several elements that have a distinctive influence on community participation in the decision making as well as in the design and implementation associated with community-based interventions. These elements include civic engagement, local leadership development, community participation, trust, skill building, transparency, and inclusiveness. Community processes typically have a sequence of activities that incorporate learning about various options available for health improvement, deliberations associated with the selection of one or more options, consideration of the appropriate methods to implement the health improvement initiatives, and critical reflection on the entire process. The way that decisions are made and carried out not only can be important to the success of a strategy or policy—and thus to community well-being—but also can have a direct impact on well-being through benefits of broad participation and buy-in to decisions (Minkler and Wallerstein, 2008; Wallerstein and Duran, 2010). Community processes also support local adaptation and implementation of community-based interventions through feedback on the successes and failures of these health improvement initiatives.

Leadership development According to Goodman and colleagues (1998), a healthy community needs diverse leadership that includes "a strong base of actively involved residents." A diverse leadership will include elected or appointed leaders (e.g., mayor or councilman) and informal leaders (e.g., opinion leaders and community activists). Cook and colleagues (2009) report that strong local leaders have been found to positively influence community vitality by, for example, securing funding to produce change in the quantity of housing. Ricketts and Ladewig (2008, p. 137), in a study of how sense of community and social capital work with leadership to encourage change, found that "community leaders assisted in developing important relationships, establishing communication and imparting community direction, thereby providing the needed link between variables."

Skill-building The skills related to community processes include those associated with the process of community organizing. A model based on work by Wechsler and Schnepp (1993) included the principles of listening, relationships, challenge, action, reflection, evaluation, and celebration in a cyclical framework that provides a map for how to build an engaged community that promotes ongoing participation in decision making related to those actions that affect the community as a whole. Individuals who have the ability to clearly communicate their values, interests, and motivations are key to this cyclical framework. They possess the essential qualities of inclusion, trustworthiness, leadership development, and self-reflection (Chavez et al., 2010).

Civic engagement or participation Active volunteers and people with high and medium civic participation (defined as belonging to one [medium] or two or more [high] clubs or organizations) report higher levels of well-being than those who are not active, and all-cause mortality rates were found to be lower in communities with high levels of civic engagement (Morrow-Howell et al., 2003; Poortinga, 2006) and "a strong institutional infrastructure for civic participation" (Lee, 2010, p. 1840). Neighborhood residents can play an important role in maintaining order in their neighborhoods when they participate in local organizations that make collective efforts possible (Skogan, 1989). Furthermore, a wide array of participation from community stakeholders can impact local government actions (Burby, 2003) and "institutions that promote participation and public discussion help citizens to make informed choices on many aspects that impinge on the QoL [quality of life]" (Stiglitz et al., 2009, p. 177).

Community mobilization Community mobilization, sometimes referred to as community organization, is the "organization and activation of a community to address local problems" (Shults et al., 2009, p. 362). Communities are complex social systems, and the process used to determine whether or not to implement potential prevention policies or strategies can, in its own right, be important to the successful implementation of the programs or policies. Shults and colleagues (2009) found that community mobilization efforts advance the problem-solving capacity and empowerment of both individuals and communities which, they said, can promote other beneficial effects. In terms of health, for example, "community mobilization is a promising approach to addressing health disparities" (Collie-Akers et al., 2009, p. 118S).

Equity Equity is an important element of community process. Being inclusive of various stakeholders contributes to equity, but inclusiveness can vary in important dimensions that may leave significant inequities in a process. A problematic inequality in community process, for example, is that some people may have more influence on decisions than others. Some stakeholders need support that improves their access to relevant evidence, but including them without support may leave important inequalities in their ability to contribute to a decision. Inequalities in the development of leadership across various groups may lead to inequalities in influence of the process of decision making about community-based interventions. More generally, even if the process is inclusive, power relationships may vary significantly and affect the way that interventions are valued, designed, and adopted.

The Problem of Double Counting

In a valuation framework with several domains such as those discussed above, the values captured in one domain should not be included again in one of the other domains—that is, they should not be double counted. Consider, for example, a case in which an intervention improves some aspect of a person's health (such as a reduction in obesity) and this improvement in turn leads the person to return to school and gain more education. It is important that the valuation of the health gain be kept independent of the valuation of the increased education. One way to approach this is for the valuation of the health gain to be done comprehensively, such that the induced effect on education (and its value) is captured in the gains attributed to the improvement in health and captured in the health domain. In this case, the education gain should not be recorded independently and included in the community well-being domain. To do so would be double counting. A second approach would be to do the valuation of the health gain narrowly, so that it is limited to direct improvements in the person's health. In this case, the induced education gain would have to be valued separately with the value included in the overall assessment as a gain in community well-being.

The following section explores the issue of assessing the resource use or costs of a community-based prevention intervention.

VALUING RESOURCES AND COSTS FOR COMMUNITY-BASED PREVENTION

Community-based prevention is a collaborative effort among three sets of actors: funders, community partners, and participants. Typically all of these actors contribute resources to the implementation of community-based interventions. As a result of an implementation, various effects are experienced by the actors as benefits, harms, savings, or costs (Drummond et al., 2005; Luce et al., 1996; Parasuraman et al., 2006). To ensure that the full range of resources used by the intervention is identified and counted, a broad net should be cast.

The funders of an intervention are those government agencies (international, federal, state, or local), private foundations, corporations, and individual philanthropists and donors that provide financial resources to the community partners to implement interventions. These funds are typically used to pay for salaries, wages, and benefits of staff, the cost of outside professionals and consultants, facilities costs (e.g., overhead, space, and equipment), program materials (e.g., devices and printed materials) and supplies. Funders provide other resources as well, such as professional expertise, consultants, training, and program materials to support community partners.

Community partners, such as local government agencies, nonprofit agencies like the YMCA or United Way, local employers, schools, churches, and physicians, are typically responsible for implementing the intervention. They provide staff, facilities, supplies, equipment, and program-related materials. Some of these resources are paid for by grants from funders. However, community partners themselves may donate additional staff time, facilities, equipment, and materials. The community partners may also use volunteer time. Volunteer time includes the unpaid services of individuals who are not employed by the community partners but who participate in the development, production, and delivery of the intervention. Community partners sometimes also incur intangible costs, such as costs associated with building coalitions and collaborations among community organizations. It is not unusual for community partners to have different organizational cultures, missions, and values. Each community partner may have to change or compromise its brand, reputation, and goals in order to participate in the community-based prevention program with a broader coalition of community partners.

Community-based prevention also requires the time and resources of participants. Participating in an intervention may reduce the time that participants can spend on work or leisure. These time costs need to be considered lest the intervention appear less costly than it really is compared to interventions that rely on participants purchasing goods or services. Some interventions may require participants to make various purchases items, such as of devices, equipment, transportation, and childcare expenses. Also, a participant's family members may have to use their time and resources to accommodate his or her participating in the intervention. Participation may also have intangible costs. The intervention may require participants to do things that they feel are unpleasant or to stop doing things that they enjoy. Sometimes these opinions about the intervention are temporary and after participants adopt the lifestyle change they prefer the new behaviors to the old ones. However, feelings about the intervention sometimes do not change.

Nonparticipants can also be impacted by the implementation of community-based prevention. The committee prefers to treat these impacts as benefits and harms rather than as savings and costs.

To determine the cost of a community-based prevention program one must first decide from whose perspective the determination is being made. Funders may consider only their program costs, while community partners may want to consider only the costs that they bear. However, a comprehensive perspective considers the costs of all of the resources expended, including those of the participants. This perspective eliminates the possibility of double counting because it looks at the resources used to provide the intervention. This perspective assumes that resources have alternative uses and therefore opportunity costs. If a resource is traded in a market place, then its opportunity costs can be estimated as its market prices, i.e., wages and salaries for personnel, rental rates for facilities, and purchase prices for equipment, services, and material. Sometimes, however, market prices may not represent the true resource costs—for example, if those prices are too high because they include excess profits or too low because of government subsidies.

The opportunity costs of non-market items such as volunteer and participant time can be estimated at an appropriate wage rate (Luce et al., 1996). The choice of a wage is left to the judgment of the analysts. Examples are actual, average, or overtime wage rates of volunteers and participants. In the case of non-working participants, the disabled, and children, using wage data is an imperfect solution, but there are no good alternatives in economic evaluation literature. Some analysts use zero in these cases, implying that there is no alternative use for volunteers' and participants' time. This assumption is unreasonable, however, given that volunteers and participants do have other uses for their time, uses that they value. Not counting volunteer and participant time misleads decision makers on the true costs of an intervention, much in the same way as overlooking the community wellness and community process aspects of community-based prevention misleads decision makers on the true benefits and harms.

As another example, the occupation of a building by a program means that the building cannot be used in another activity—the intervention has eliminated this alternative use. From an economic perspective, the cost of using the building is the value of the services that the building would have generated in this alternative use. Even if the program pays no rent, there is still a cost, and that cost can be approximated by the rents paid for similar buildings.

The valuation of an intervention is based on the changes in outcomes and in resources used that were caused by an intervention, as compared to an alternative. The alternative can be the existing situation (sometimes called the *status quo*) or another intervention. If an intervention uses less of some resources than the alternative, it yields savings for those items of cost. Sometimes the total costs of an intervention may be less than those of the alternative, yielding an overall saving. The crucial point is that savings become apparent only when two alternatives are compared and that the savings depend on the specific comparison. An intervention that yields savings, i.e., uses fewer resources, compared to one alternative may not yield savings when compared to a different alternative.

For example, in addition to the costs of implementing an intervention, community-based prevention may reduce costs in health care and other social service sectors of the community. For example, a community health workers program that helps residents with chronic health conditions improve their self-care and medication use could result in lower emergency room use and rates of preventable hospitalizations. This lowers the residents' hospital care costs, thus generating savings for them and their health plans. Another example is community-based prevention targeting at-risk youth who have a dual diagnosis of mental illness and substance abuse. In addition to helping youth maintain their mental health and staying drug free, such a program could reduce costs in the juvenile justice system through lower arrest and incarceration rates. These types of cost offsets should be considered when computing the costs of community-based prevention. The cost offsets should not be confused with the benefits of the programs, which are improvements in health, community well-being, and community process.

Table 3-1 provides a hypothetical example of a total costs computation for an illustrative community-based renovation of a derelict park undertaken to promote physical activity among the town's citizens. Donated resources are valued according to the closest market rates for time, space, and other goods and services. The total net costs are $10,000.

TABLE 3-1 Hypothetical Community-Based Renovation of a Park: Cost Computation

Type of Costs	Park Left as Is, No Exercise Facilities	Park Renovated with Exercise Facilities	Difference
Intervention Costs			
Donated time and space for meetings to plan renovation	0	$50,000	$50,000
Purchased plants, equipment	0	$100,000	$100,000
Park renovation and maintenance paid by town (includes state grant)	$10,000	$50,000	$40,000
Donated time for park renovation and maintenance	0	$10,000	$10,000
Donated time to lead exercise activities	0	$10,000	$10,000
Cost Offsets			
Town citizens' health care costs	$1,000,000	$850,000	–$150,000
Town juvenile justice costs	$200,000	$150,000	–$50,000
TOTAL COSTS	$1,210,000	1, 220,000	$10,000

Resource use and benefits occur over a period of time that may extend many years into the future. If that period is greater than 1 year, it is appropriate to discount, in order to capture two realities: people prefer benefits sooner rather than later; and resources are productive—if they are not consumed now but are invested instead, they will produce even more resources in the future. (It is important to note that the concept of a discount rate is net of and different from that of inflation.) In cost–benefit and cost-effectiveness analysis, the practice is to discount both costs and benefits and to discount them at the same rate (Lipscomb et al., 1996; OMB, 2003). When the time horizon is very long, it can lead to difficult questions regarding discounting. This is particularly true of prevention interventions where the costs accrue immediately but the benefits accrue much later. In theory this could lead to an undervaluation of the long-term benefits relative to the short-term costs. In this case it is important to value the long-term benefits adequately rather than attempt to adjust the discount rate (IOM, 2006b; Lipscomb et al., 1996).

Various governmental and nongovernmental groups recommend—or require—specific discount rates, but there is no general agreement among them on what the discount rate should be (Jawad and Ozbay, 2006). For example, the Office of Management and Budget recommends a real (adjusted for inflation) discount rate of 7 percent per year, with 3 percent as an alternative to test the sensitivity of an evaluation's results to the discount rate (OMB, 2003). The Panel on Cost-Effectiveness in Health and Medicine recommends a real rate of 3 percent for cost-effectiveness analyses and the National Institute of Health and Clinical Excellence in the United Kingdom requires a real rate of 3.5 percent.

DATA SOURCES AND INDICATORS FOR
VALUING COMMUNITY-BASED PREVENTION

There are a variety of sources of data on health, including surveys (e.g., the National Health Interview Survey and the Behavioral Risk Factor Surveillance System), cohort studies (e.g., the Framingham Heart Study), registries, health services data, vital statistics, and data collected by state public health agencies. Unfortunately, there are several limitations on using these data for local, community-based measurement (IOM, 2011b). For example, national surveys are unable to provide the detailed data needed for local estimates without specifically designing local data collection. Registries and health services data provide information only about those who seek and receive health services, cohort studies are resource intensive, and vital statistics are subject to coding errors (IOM, 2011b). To collect information to measure baseline health and changes in health at the local level may require developing and implementing local surveys aimed at the specific health issues of interest.

Identifying measures and sources of information for community well-being and community process elements is even more challenging than collecting such information about health. Table 3-2 lists elements and indicators that could be used in the three domains of interest: health, community well-being, and community process. As stated before, these are examples only. The actual elements and indicators chosen will depend on the community-based prevention intervention being considered.

Applying methods from systems science to community-based prevention efforts can help increase our understanding of the complex interrelationships among factors important to building healthy populations and healthy communities. The following chapter discusses how a framework for valuing resides within a decision-making context, reviews eight frameworks currently used to assess community-based prevention, and discusses the strengths and limitations of each for addressing the special characteristics of community-based prevention.

TABLE 3-2 Domains and Examples of Elements and Indicators for Valuing Community-Based Prevention Interventions

Value Component	Elements (examples)	Possible Measures (data sources)
Health	*Overall* 1. Quality of life 2. Perceived health	*Overall* 1. Quality-adjusted life year (QALY) or health-adjusted life expectancy (HALE) 2. Self-reported health status
	Physical 1. Mortality (overall and per cause) 2. Morbidity 3. Functional capability 4. Injuries	*Physical* 1. Deaths 2. Rates of conditions or diseases of interest, unhealthy days 3. Level of activities of daily living, exercise 4. Rates of injuries
	Mental 1. Cognition 2. Morbidity 3. Depression Anxiety Stress Perceived well-being 4. Suicide rates	*Mental—Change in rates* 1. Cognitive Abilities Screening Instrument (Adult), Dementia Rating Scale (Adult), Differential Abilities Scale (Children) 2. Self-reported unhealthy days mental 3. Self-reported healthy days mental 4. Rates of suicides
Community Well-Being	*Built environment* 1. Land use 2. Transportation 3. Building quality (indoor air) 4. Food systems	*Built environment* 1. Number and quality of facilities—schools, libraries, housing 2. Number of sidewalks for walking, bike paths, buses, metro/trains, automobiles. 3. Levels of pollutants (e.g., radon, tobacco smoke, chemicals) 4. Grocery stores with healthy choices, farmer's markets

continued

TABLE 3-2   Continued

Value Component	Elements (examples)	Possible Measures (data sources)
	Natural physical environment Green space	*Natural physical environment* Parks, preserved open spaces, beauty

	Social and economic environments
	1. Social support and social networks
	2. Social cohesion
	3. Education
	   a. Resources
	
	   b. Achievement
	
	   c. Health literacy
	
	4. Employment
	   a. Safe work places
	
	   b. Stress
	
	   c. Income
	5. Crime/safety
	6. Access to health care and health insurance
		Social and economic environments
		1. Number, type, frequency of contact
		2. Trust, respect
		3. Number and quality of schools
		   a. Books, computers, play equipment, class size
		   b. 3rd-grade reading level, high school and college graduation rates
		   c. Change in level of health literacy
		4. Employment/unemployment rate
		   a. Physical environment and job effort
		   b. Job demand versus control, job effort versus rewards
		   c. Wages, food stamp use
		5. Rates for various crimes
		6. Number and type of health care facilities, rate of uninsured

Community Process	1. Local leadership development 2. Skill building 3. Civic engagement or participation 4. Community mobilization	1. Elected leaders reflect community diversity, number and type of community activists 2. Number and type of peer counselors and community organizers 3. Voting rates, volunteering, participation in clubs or other local organizations 4. Involvement in civic activities (e.g., town hall meetings)

REFERENCES

AHRQ (Agency for Healthcare Research and Quality). 2012. *2011 national healthcare quality & disparities reports.* Rockville, MD: Agency for Healthcare Research and Quality.

APHA (American Public Health Association). No date. *Health disparities: The basics.* http://www.apha.org/NR/rdonlyres/54C4CC4D-E86D-479A-BABB-5D42B3FDC8BD/0/Hlth-Disparty_Primer_FINAL.pdf (accessed June 29, 2012).

Barakat-Haddad, C., S. J. Elliott, and D. Pengelly. 2012. Health impacts of air pollution: A life course approach for examining predictors of respiratory health in adulthood. *Annals of Epidemiology* 22(4):239-249.

Barnett, W. S. 1985. *The Perry Preschool Program and its long-term effects: A benefit-cost analysis.* Ypsilanti, MI: High/Scope Educational Research Foundation.

Barnett, W. S. 1996. *Lives in the balance: Benefit-cost analysis of the Perry Preschool Program through age 27.* Ypsilanti, MI: High/Scope Educational Research Foundation.

Berkman, L., and T. A. Glass. 2000. Social integration, social networks, social support, and health. In *Social epidemiology,* edited by L. Berkman and I. Kawachi. New York: Oxford University Press. Pp. 137-173.

Berkman, L., and I. Kawachi. 2000. *Social epidemiology.* New York: Oxford University Press.

Besser, L. M., and A. L. Dannenberg. 2005. Walking to public transit: Steps to help meet physical activity recommendations. *American Journal of Preventive Medicine* 29(4):273-280.

Bodor, J., J. Rice, T. Farley, C. Swalm, and D. Rose. 2010. The association between obesity and urban food environments. *Journal of Urban Health* 87(5):771-781.

BSSR/NIH (Office of Behavioral and Social Sciences Research and National Institutes of Health). 2012. *Dissemination and implementation.* http://obssr.od.nih.gov/scientific_areas/translation/dissemination_and_implementation/index.aspx (accessed March 15, 2012).

Burby, R. J. 2003. Making plans that matter. *Journal of the American Planning Association* 69(1):33.

Carlson, D., R. Haveman, T. Kaplan, and B. Wolfe. 2011. The benefits and costs of the Section 8 housing subsidy program: A framework and estimates of first-year effects. *Journal of Policy Analysis and Management* 30(2):233-255.

Carroll, C., M. Patterson, S. Wood, A. Booth, J. Rick, and S. Balain. 2007. A conceptual framework for implementation fidelity. *Implementation Science* 2:40.

Catalano, R. A., S. L. Lind, A. B. Rosenblatt, and C. C. Attkisson. 1999. Unemployment and foster home placements: estimating the net effect of provocation and inhibition. *American Journal of Public Health* 89(6):851-855.

CDC (Centers for Disease Control and Prevention). 2012a. *Communities putting prevention to work.* http://www.cdc.gov/CommunitiesPuttingPreventiontoWork (accessed March 15, 2012).

CDC. 2012b. *Community transformation grants.* http://www.cdc.gov/communitytransformation/ (accessed March 15, 2012).

Chavez, V., M. Minkler, N. Wallerstein, and M. S. Spencer. 2010. Community organizing for health and social justice. In *Prevention is primary.* 2nd ed, edited by L. Cohen, V. Chavez and S. Chehimi. San Francisco: Jossey-Bass. Pp. 95-119.

Cohen, S., I. Brissette, D. P. Skoner, and W. J. Doyle. 2000. Social integration and health: The case of the common cold. *Journal of Social Structure* 1(3):1-7.

Collie-Akers, V., J. A. Schultz, V. Carson, S. B. Fawcett, and M. Ronan. 2009. REACH 2010: Kansas City, Missouri. *Health Promotion Practice* 10(2 Suppl):118S-127S.

Cook, C. C., S. R. Crull, M. J. Bruin, B. L. Yust, M. C. Shelley, S. Laux, J. Memken, S. Niemeyer, and B. White. 2009. Evidence of a housing decision chain in rural community vitality. *Rural Sociology* 74(1):113-137.

Coombes, E., A. P. Jones, and M. Hillsdon. 2010. The relationship of physical activity and overweight to objectively measured green space accessibility and use. *Social Science and Medicine* 70(6):816-822.

Cornwell, E. Y., and L. J. Waite. 2009. Social disconnectedness, perceived isolation, and health among older adults. *Journal of Health and Social Behavior* 50(1):31-48.

Cradock, A. L., I. Kawachi, G. A. Colditz, S. L. Gortmaker, and S. L. Buka. 2009. Neighborhood social cohesion and youth participation in physical activity in Chicago. *Social Science and Medicine* 68(3):427.

de Nazelle, A., M. J. Nieuwenhuijsen, J. M. Anto, M. Brauer, D. Briggs, C. Braun-Fahrlander, N. Cavill, A. R. Cooper, H. Desqueyroux, S. Fruin, G. Hoek, L. I. Panis, N. Janssen, M. Jerrett, M. Joffe, Z. J. Andersen, E. van Kempen, S. Kingham, N. Kubesch, K. M. Leyden, J. D. Marshall, J. Matamala, G. Mellios, M. Mendez, H. Nassif, D. Ogilvie, R. Peiro, K. Perez, A. Rabl, M. Ragletti, D. Rodriguez, D. Rojas, P. Ruiz, J. F. Sallis, J. Terwoert, J. F. Toussaint, J. Tuomisto, M. Zuurbier, E. Lebret. 2011. Improving health through policies that promote active travel: A review of evidence to support integrated health impact assessment. *Environment International* (37)4:766-777.

Drummond, M., M. Schulper, G. Torrance, B. Obrien, and G. Stoddart. 2005. *Methods for economic evaluation of health care programmes*, 3rd ed. New York: Oxford University Press Inc.

Ellaway, A., S. Macintyre, and X. Bonnefoy. 2005. Graffiti, greenery, and obesity in adults: Secondary analysis of European cross sectional survey. *BMJ* 331(7517):611-612.

Eller, M., R. Holle, R. Landgraf, and A. Mielck. 2008. Social network effect on self-rated health in type 2 diabetic patients—results from a longitudinal population-based study. *International Journal of Public Health* 53(4):188-194.

EPA (Environmental Protection Agency). 2001. *Healthy buildings, healthy people: A vision for the 21st century*. Washington, DC: EPA.

Ewing, R., R. C. Brownson, and D. Berrigan. 2006. Relationship between urban sprawl and weight of United States youth. *American Journal of Preventive Medicine* 31(6):464-474.

Frumkin, H. 2003. Healthy places: Exploring the evidence. *American Journal of Public Health* 93(9):1451-1456.

Garnefski, N., and R. Diekstra. 1996. Perceived social support from family, school, and peers: Relationship with emotional and behavioral problems among adolescents. *Journal of the American Academy of Child and Adolescent Psychiatry* 35(12):1657-1664.

Glasgow, R., T. Vogt, and S. Boles. 1999. Evaluating the public health impact of health promotion interventions: The RE-AIM framework. *American Journal of Public Health* 89(9):1322-1327.

Goodman, R. M., M. A. Speers, K. McLeroy, S. Fawcett, M. Kegler, E. Parker, S. R. Smith, T. D. Sterling, and N. Wallerstein. 1998. Identifying and defining the dimensions of community capacity to provide a basis for measurement. *Health Education and Behavior* 25(3):258-278.

Gorey, K. M. 2001. Early childhood education: A meta-analytic affirmation of the short- and long-term benefits of educational opportunity. *School Psychology Quarterly* 16(1):9-30.

Green, L. W. 1986. The theory of participation: A qualitative analysis of its expression in national and international health policies. *Advances in Health Education and Promotion* 1:211-236.

Haan, P., and M. Myck. 2009. *Dynamics of poor health and non-employment*: Bonn, Germany: Forschungsinst zur Zukunft der Arbeit.

Hammond, R. A. 2009. Complex systems modeling for obesity research. *Preventing Chronic Disease* 6(3):A97.

Hanleybrown, F., J. Kania, and M. Kramer. 2012. Channeling change: Making collective impact work. *Stanford Social Innovation Review*. http://www.ssireview.org/pdf/Channeling_Change_PDF.pdf (accessed July 30, 2012).

Harrison, R. A., I. Gemmell, and R. F. Heller. 2007. The population effect of crime and neighbourhood on physical activity: An analysis of 15,461 adults. *Journal of Epidemiology and Community Health* 61(1):34-39.

Hirschfield, A., and K. J. Bowers. 1997. The effect of social cohesion on levels of recorded crime in disadvantaged areas. *Urban Studies* 34(8):1275-1295.

Homer, J., and G. Hirsch. 2006. System dynamics modeling for public health: Background and opportunities. *American Journal of Public Health* 96:452-458.

Horowitz, C., M. Robinson, and S. Seifer. 2009. Community-based participatory research from the margin to the mainstream: Are researchers prepared? *Circulation* 119:2633-2642.

Huang, T. T., A. Drewnosksi, S. Kumanyika, and T. A. Glass. 2009. A systems-oriented multilevel framework for addressing obesity in the 21st century. *Preventing Chronic Disease* 6(3):A82.

IOM (Institute of Medicine). 2001. *Rebuilding the unity of health and the environment: A new vision of environmental health for the 21st Century*. Washington, DC: National Academy Press.

IOM. 2003. *Unequal treatment: Confronting racial and ethnic disparities in health care.* Washington, DC: The National Academies Press.

IOM. 2006a. *Genes, behavior, and the social environment.* Washington, DC: The National Academies Press.

IOM. 2006b. *Valuing health for regulatory cost-effectiveness analysis.* Washington, DC: The National Academies Press.

IOM. 2009. *State of the USA health indicators.* Washington, DC: The National Academies Press.

IOM. 2010. *Bridging the evidence gap in obesity prevention: A framework to inform decision making.* Washington, DC: The National Academies Press.

IOM. 2011a. *Climate hange, the indoor environment, and health.* Washington, DC: The National Academies Press.

IOM. 2011b. *A nationwide framework for surveillance of cardiovascular and chronic lung diseases.* Washington, DC: The National Academies Press.

Jawad, D., and K. Ozbay. 2006. *The discount rate in life cycle cost analysis of transportation projects.* Paper read at Annual Meeting of the Transportation Research Board, January 22-26, Washington, DC. http://rits.rutgers.edu/files/discountrate_lifecycle.pdf.

Jin, R. L., C. P. Shah, and T. J. Svoboda. 1995. The impact of unemployment on health: A review of the evidence. *Canadian Medical Association Journal* 153(5):529-540.

Johnson, S. L., B. S. Solomon, W. C. Shields, E. M. McDonald, L. B. McKenzie, and A. C. Gielen. 2009. Neighborhood violence and its association with mothers' health: Assessing the relative importance of perceived safety and exposure to violence. *Journal of Urban Health* 86(4):538-550.

Kania, J., and M. Kramer. 2011. Collective impact. *Stanford Social Innovation Review* Winter:36-41. http://www.ssireview.org/pdf/2011_WI_Feature_Kania.pdf (accessed July 30, 2012).

Kawachi, I., and L. Berkman. 2003. *Neighborhoods and health*. New York: Oxford University Press.

Keane, C. 1998. Evaluating the influence of fear of crime as an environmental mobility restrict or on women's routine activities. *Environment and Behavior* 30(1):60-74.

Kim, D., S. V. Subramanian, and I. Kawachi. 2008. Social capital and physical health: A systematic review of the literature. In *Social capital and health*, edited by I. Kawachi, S. V. Subramanian, and D. Kim. New York: Springer. Pp. 139-190.

Lachapelle, U., and L. D. Frank. 2009. Transit and health: Mode of transport, employer-sponsored public transit pass programs, and physical activity. *Journal of Public Health Policy*:S73-S94.

Lee, M. R. 2010. The protective effects of civic communities against all-cause mortality. *Social Science and Medicine* 70(11):1840-1846.

Leung, C. W., B. A. Laraia, M. Kelly, D. Nickleach, N. E. Adler, L. H. Kushi, and I. H. Yen. 2011. The influence of neighborhood food stores on change in young girls' body mass index. *American Journal of Preventive Medicine* 41(1):43-51.

Lindén-Boström, M., C. Persson, and C. Eriksson. 2010. Neighbourhood characteristics, social capital and self-rated health—a population-based survey in Sweden. *BMC Public Health* 10(1):628.

Linnan, L., and A. Steckler. 2002. Process evaluation for public health interventions and research: An overview. In *Process evaluation for public health interventions and research*, edited by A. Steckler and L. Linnan. San Francisco: Jossey-Bass. Pp. 1-24.

Lipscomb, J., M. C. Weinstein, and G. W. Torrance. 1996. Time preference. In *Cost-effectiveness in health and medicine*, edited by M. R. Gold, J. E. Siegel, L. B. Russell, and M. C. Weinstein. New York: Oxford University Press.

Livingood, W. C., J. P. Allegrante, C. O. Airhihenbuwa, N. M. Clark, R. C. Windsor, M. A. Zimmerman, and L. W. Green. 2011. Applied social and behavioral science to address complex health problems. *American Journal of Preventive Medicine* 41(5):525-531.

Lleras-Muney, A. 2005. The relationship between education and adult mortality in the United States. *Review of Economic Studies* 72(1):189-221.

Lopez, R. 2004. Urban sprawl and risk for being overweight or obese. *American Journal of Public Health* 94(9):1574-1579.

Luce, B., W. Manning, J. Siegel, and J. Lipscomb. 1996. Estimating costs in cost-effectiveness analysis. In *Cost effectiveness in health and medicine*, edited by M. Gold and J. Siegel. New York: Oxford University Press.

Luke, D., and K. Stamatakis. 2012. Systems science methods in public health: Dynamics, networks, and agents. *Annual Review of Public Health* 33:357-376.

Maas, J., R. A. Verheij, P. P. Groenewegen, S. De Vries, and P. Spreeuwenberg. 2006. Green space, urbanity, and health: How strong is the relation? *Journal of Epidemiology and Community Health* 60(7):587-592.

Maas, J., R. A. Verheij, S. de Vries, P. Spreeuwenberg, F. G. Schellevis, and P. P. Groenewegen. 2009. Morbidity is related to a green living environment. *Journal of Epidemiology and Community Health* 63(12):967-973.

Mabry, P., D. Olster, G. Morgan, and D. Abrams. 2008. Interdisciplinarity and systems science to improve population health: A view from the NIH Office of Behavioral and Social Sciences Research. *American Journal of Preventive Medicine* 35(Suppl):S211-S224.

Mabry, P. L., S. E. Marcus, P. I. Clark, S. J. Leischow, and D. Méndez. 2010. Systems science: A revolution in public health policy research. *American Journal of Public Health* 100(7):1161-1163.

MacDonald, J. M., R. J. Stokes, D. A. Cohen, A. Kofner, and G. K. Ridgeway. 2010. The effect of light rail transit on body mass index and physical activity. *American Journal of Preventive Medicine* 39(2):105-112.

Madon, T., K. Hofman, L. Kupfer, and R. Glass. 2007. Implementation science. *Science* 318:1728-1729.

Malecki, C. K., and M. K. Demaray. 2007. Social behavior assessment and response to intervention. *Handbook of Response to Intervention*:161-171.

Marmot, M. G., and R. G. Wilkinson. 1999. *Social determinants of health*. Oxford: Oxford University Press.

Maulik, P. K., W. W. Eaton, and C. P. Bradshaw. 2009. The role of social network and support in mental health service use: Findings from the Baltimore ECA study. *Psychiatric Services* 60(9):1222-1229.

McPherson, E. G., D. Nowak, G. Heisler, S. Grimmond, C. Souch, R. Grant, and R. Rowntree. 1997. Quantifying urban forest structure, function, and value: The Chicago urban forest climate project. *Urban Ecosystems* 1(1):49-61.

Meadows, D. 1999. *Leverage points: Places to intervene in a system.* Hartland, VT: Sustainability Institute. http://www.sustainer.org/pubs/Leverage_Points.pdf (accessed May 19, 2012).

Michimi, A., and M. C. Wimberly. 2010. Associations of supermarket accessibility with obesity and fruit and vegetable consumption in the conterminous United States. *International Journal of Health Geographics* 9(1):49.

Milam, A. J., C. D. M. Furr-Holden, and P. J. Leaf. 2010. Perceived school and neighborhood safety, neighborhood violence and academic achievement in urban school children. *Urban Review* 42(5):458-467.

Minkler, M., and N. Wallerstein. 2008. *Community based participatory research for health: From process to outcomes.* San Francisco: Jossey Bass.

Minkler, M., V. B. Vásquez, M. Tajik, and D. Petersen. 2008. Promoting environmental justice through community-based participatory research: The role of community and partnership capacity. *Health Education & Behavior* 35(1):119-137.

Morland, K., A. V. Diez Roux, and S. Wing. 2006. Supermarkets, other food stores, and obesity: The Atherosclerosis Risk in Communities Study. *American Journal of Preventive Medicine* 30(4):333-339.

Morrow-Howell, N., J. Hinterlong, P. A. Rozario, and F. Tang. 2003. Effects of volunteering on the well-being of older adults. *Journals of Gerontology Series B: Psychological Sciences and Social Sciences* 58(3):S137-S145.

Nelson, M. C., P. Gordon-Larsen, Y. Song, and B. M. Popkin. 2006. Built and social environments: Associations with adolescent overweight and activity. *American Journal of Preventive Medicine* 31(2):109-117.

NHLBI/NIH (National Heart, Lung, and Blood Institute and National Institutes of Health). 2012. Division for the Application of Research Discoveries. http://www.nhlbi.nih.gov/about/dard/index.htm (accessed March 15, 2012).

OMB (Office of Management and Budget). 2003. *Circular A-4.* http://www.whitehouse.gov/omb/circulars_a004_a4 (accessed June 14, 2012).

Parasuraman, S., C. Salvador, and K. Frick. 2006. Measuring economic outcomes. In *Economic evaluation in U.S. health care: Principles and applications,* edited by L. Pizzi and J. Lofland. Sudbury, MA: Jones and Bartlett. Pp. 15-35.

Patton, M. 2002. *Qualitative research and evaluation methods,* 3rd ed. Thousand Oaks, CA: Sage.

Poortinga, W. 2006. Social relations or social capital? Individual and community health effects of bonding social capital. *Social Science and Medicine* 63(1):255-270.

Powell, L. M., M. C. Auld, F. J. Chaloupka, P. M. O'Malley, and L. D. Johnston. 2007. Associations between access to food stores and adolescent body mass index. *American Journal of Preventive Medicine* 33(4):S301-S307.

Raphael, S., and R. Winter-Ebmer. 2001. Identifying the effect of unemployment on crime. *Journal of Law and Economics* 44(1):259-283.

Ricketts, K. G., and H. Ladewig. 2008. A path analysis of community leadership within viable rural communities in Florida. *Leadership* 4(2):137-157.

Ross, C. E., and S. J. Jang. 2000. Neighborhood disorder, fear, and mistrust: The buffering role of social ties with neighbors. *American Journal of Community Psychology* 28(4):401-420.

Rossi, P., M. Lipsey, and H. Freeman. 2004. *Evaluation: A systematic approach*. Thousand Oaks: Sage Publications, Inc.

Rueda, S., L. Chambers, M. Wilson, C. Mustard, S. B. Rourke, A. Bayoumi, J. Raboud, and J. Lavis. 2012. Association of returning to work with better health in working-aged adults: A systematic review. *American Journal of Public Health* 102(3):541-556.

RWJF (Robert Wood Johnson Founation). 2012. *Healthy kids, healthy communities*. http://www.healthykidshealthycommunities.org/ (accessed March 15, 2012).

Saha, S., U. G. Gerdtham, and P. Johansson. 2010. Economic evaluation of lifestyle interventions for preventing diabetes and cardiovascular diseases. *International Journal of Environmental Research and Public Health* 7(8):3150-3195.

Sandoval, J. A., J. Lucero, J. Oetzel, M. Avila, L. Belone, M. Mau, C. Pearson, G. Tafoya, B. Duran, and L. I. Rios. 2012. Process and outcome constructs for evaluating community-based participatory research projects: A matrix of existing measures. *Health Education Research* 27(4):680-690.

Schweinhart, L. J., H. V. Barnes, and D. P. Weikart. 1993. *Significant benefits: The High/Scope Perry Preschool Study through age 27*. Ypsilanti, MI: High/Scope Educational Research Foundation.

Shareck, M., and A. Ellaway. 2011. Neighbourhood crime and smoking: The role of objective and perceived crime measures. *BMC Public Health* 11(1):930.

Shimizu, H. 2011. Social cohesion and self-sacrificing behavior. *Public Choice* 149(3):427-440.

Shults, R. A., R. W. Elder, J. L. Nichols, D. A. Sleet, R. Compton, and S. K. Chattopadhyay. 2009. Effectiveness of multicomponent programs with community mobilization for reducing alcohol-impaired driving. *American Journal of Preventive Medicine* 37(4):360-371.

Skogan, W. G. 1989. Communities, crime, and neighborhood organization. *Crime & Delinquency* 35(3):437-457.

Stanley, D. 2003. What do we know about social cohesion: The research perspective of the federal government's social cohesion research network. *Canadian Journal of Sociology* 28(1):5-17.

Stansfeld, S., J. Head, and J. Ferrie. 1999. Short-term disability, sickness absence, and social gradients in the Whitehall II study. *International Journal of Law and Psychiatry* 22(5-6):425-439.

Sterman, J. 2000. *Business dynamics. Systems thinking and modeling for a complex world*. Boston: McGraw-Hill.

Stiglitz, J. E., A. Sen, and J. Fitoussi. 2009. *Report by the Commission on the Measurement of Economic Performance and Social Progress*. http://www.stiglitz-sen-fitoussi.fr/documents/rapport_anglais.pdf (accessed July 30, 2012).

Strully, K. 2009. Job loss and health in the U.S. labor market. *Demography* 46(2):221-246.

Teddlie, C., and A. Tashakkori. 2009. *Foundations of mixed methods research: Integrating quantititative and qualitative approaches in the social and behavioral sciences*. Thousand Oaks, CA: Sage.

TRB/IOM (Transportation Research Board and Institute of Medicine). 2005. *Does the built environment influence physical activity? Examining the evidence—special report 282*. Washington, DC: The National Academies Press.

Trickett, E. J. 2009. Multilevel community-based culturally situated interventions and community impact: An ecological perspective. *American Journal of Community Psychology* 43(3):257-266.

Ulin, P., E. Robinson, and E. Tolley. 2005. *Qualitative methods in public health: A field guide for applied research*. San Francisco: Jossey-Bass.

Ulrich, R. S. 1984. View through a window may influence recovery from surgery. *Science* 224(4647):420-421.

Ulrich, W. 2000. Reflective practice in the civil society: The contribution of critically systemic thinking. *Reflective Practice* 1(2):247-268.

Van Den Berg, A. E., J. Maas, R. A. Verheij, and P. P. Groenewegen. 2010. Green space as a buffer between stressful life events and health. *Social Science and Medicine* 70(8):1203-1210.

Viswanathan, M., A. Ammerman, E. Eng, G. Garlehner, K. N. Lohr, D. Griffith, S. Rhodes, C. Samuel-Hodge, S. Maty, L. Lux, L. Webb, S. F. Sutton, T. Swinson, A. Jackman, and L. Whitener. 2004. Community-based participatory research: Assessing the evidence. *Evidence Report/Technology Assessment*(99):1-8.

Wallerstein, N., and B. Duran. 2010. Community-based participatory research contributions to intervention research: The intersection of science and practice to improve health equity. *American Journal of Public Health* 100(S1):S40-S46.

Wechsler, R., and T. Schnepp. 1993. *Community organizing for the prevention of problems related to alcohol and other drugs.* Rockville, MD: The Department of Justice, National Institute of Justice.

Weinstein, A., and P. Schimek. 2005. *How much do Americans walk? An analysis of the 2001 NHTS.* Paper read at Transportation Research Board 84th Annual Meeting, Washington, DC, January 10.

Weisbrod, G., and A. Reno. 2009. *Economic impact of public transportation investment*: American Public Transportation Association.

Wener, R. E., and G. W. Evans. 2007. A morning stroll. *Environment and Behavior* 39(1):62-74.

White, L., and S. J. Rogers. 2000. Economic circumstances and family outcomes: A review of the 1990s. *Journal of Marriage and Family* 62(4):1035-1051.

Wilkinson, R. G., and M. Marmot. 2003. *Social determinants of health: The solid facts.* Copenhagen: World Health Organization.

Wood, L., L. D. Frank, and B. Giles-Corti. 2010. Sense of community and its relationship with walking and neighborhood design. *Social Science & Medicine* 70(9):1381-1390.

4

Existing Frameworks

This chapter reviews eight frameworks that are currently used to assess the value of community-based prevention: benefit–cost analysis, cost-effectiveness analysis, Congressional Budget Office scoring, PRECEDE–PROCEED, RE-AIM, health impact assessment, the Community Preventive Services Task Force (CPSTF) guidelines, and the Canadian Health Services Research (Lomas) Model. The committee concluded that existing frameworks are inadequate for assessing the value of community-based prevention because none meet all of the most important criteria outlined in Chapter 3 and this chapter. Most lack community well-being measures other than health, some do not assess the value of the community processes by which prevention activities are planned and undertaken, many do not consider costs, and some do not give sufficient attention to the individual community context.

WHAT IS A FRAMEWORK FOR ASSESSING VALUE?

The committee concluded that a *framework for assessing value* is a structure for gathering and processing information to aid intelligent decision making and, more specifically, to help decide whether an activity or intervention is worthwhile. (Frameworks for implementation are different: They focus on how best to implement a program. See Chapter 2 for a description of the most important frameworks for the implementation of community-based prevention.)

A framework for assessing value can aid decision making by

- requiring that goals be stated clearly;
- integrating incomplete and sometimes conflicting information and beliefs;
- avoiding decision making based on arbitrary impressions or self-interest;
- clarifying trade-offs;
- promoting transparency; and
- exposing legitimate sources of disagreement and helping to work through them.

Frameworks for assessing value can be geared toward prospective or retrospective assessments of value. A prospective assessment of value is performed before an intervention takes place and is designed to help policy makers decide whether to undertake the intervention. An example of a prospective assessment is a cost estimate produced by the Congressional Budget Office. Program evaluations are concurrent or retrospective assessments of value: What can the evaluators say about an intervention's value while it is being implemented or after it has occurred? (Stufflebeam, 1999). Benefit–cost analysis, cost-effectiveness analysis, and some other valuation frameworks, may be either prospective or retrospective (Nash et al., 1975).

The committee concluded that a framework for assessing value should include the following elements:

- **A decision-making context**
  - o Who are the decision makers, what are the decisions they are making, and what are the formal and informal mechanisms by which assessments of value feed into the decision-making process?
- **A list of valued outcomes**
  - o What does the user of the framework care about? What should the user of the framework care about?
- **A list of admissible sources of evidence**
  - o What information does the user of the framework use to build the model of causation that links interventions to valued outcomes?
- **A method for weighting and summarizing**
  - o How is information on all the valued outcomes boiled down and made digestible for decision makers?

A Framework for Assessing Value Is Embedded
Within a Decision-Making Context

Frameworks have evolved to feed into specific decision-making contexts. Examples of decision-making contexts include Congress deciding whether to enact a piece of legislation, a local health department deciding how to allocate its budget to specific health promotion activities, and a community group deciding whether to organize its volunteers to undertake a specific health-related project. A framework that is appropriate and helpful in one decision-making context may not be helpful in another. As a result, the description of a framework must take into account the decision-making context in which it is or will be used.

Different decision makers come from different perspectives and emphasize different factors. Possible factors to consider include legal and ethical issues, the nature of the condition, resource availability, administrative factors, and idiosyncratic factors. These can sometimes be taken into account in the valuation framework. At other times, decision makers must consider them outside of—and in addition to—the assessment of value.

For example, while family-planning activities are legal and may be a valued outcome, they can be constrained by ethical attitudes toward abortion and contraception. Differing ethical and religious views in the community may need to be considered outside the valuation framework. The nature of the health condition may also need to be considered separately from valuation. Some conditions, such as conditions that affect young children, may evoke more sympathy and a greater sense of urgency than others.

Another factor that may need to be considered separately from the valuation is resource availability. Lack of the right resources may interfere with the adoption of an intervention, even when its assessed value is high relative to its costs; the right facilities and people may not be available. The availability of administrative mechanisms that can enhance the acceptability of an intervention is another factor that is considered in decision making but that is outside the valuing framework. For example, the Supplemental Nutrition Assistance Program (SNAP, formerly the Food Stamp Program), with its eligibility requirements to assure that benefits reach the intended population, could serve as the administrative base of a community intervention to improve the nutrition of low-income people. Finally, idiosyncratic factors, such as powerful advocates or vested interests, can outweigh assessments of value that the larger community places on interventions.

All of these factors must be taken into account in actual decisions. A framework for valuation provides a way of focusing attention on the valued outcomes and costs of interventions in a systematic way and helps make those outcomes and costs clear to the larger community in a way that promotes better choices.

A Framework Includes a List of Valued Outcomes

To provide effective support for decision making it is critical to list all the valued outcomes and to show, perhaps in a table, how much each intervention contributes to each outcome. That means that there must be some measure of how each outcome is affected by the intervention. For example, health might be measured in years of life gained or quality-adjusted life years gained. Community participation might be measured by the number of people who attend events or the hours of work volunteered in a year. Reductions in crime or in health risk factors might be represented by the statistics already established by police systems or by disease registries or health surveys.

If decision makers are choosing among a number of possible interventions, it helps if measures of valued outcomes can be devised that work across interventions so that the outcomes of the different interventions can be compared. That is, it helps if each health outcome can be measured in the same way for all interventions, if each community process outcome can be measured in the same way for all interventions, and so on. If each program has its own measures that are different from those of every other, it becomes more difficult to compare interventions.

Program costs (i.e., the value of the resources used) should also be measured. All resources should be measured, whether or not they are purchased. The time donated by community volunteers is a major example of a resource used in community-based programs, often in large quantities, that is rarely counted as a cost when choices are evaluated. The true cost of volunteer time, as with any other resource, is that if it is used for one program, it is not then available for other programs or for other activities that the volunteer might engage in. So the program chosen should be a worthwhile use of that time, preferably the best use.

A Framework Includes a List of Sources of Evidence and a Standard for Admissible Evidence

Every assessment of value is built on a model of causation, i.e., a theory of how the world works. Those models of causation can be built up from many different sources and types of evidence. Some frameworks make explicit the sources of evidence that are taken into consideration and the standards that each source of evidence must meet. The *Community Preventive Services Guide*, for example, includes a clear description of the sources from which the task force draws evidence and the standards that are used to grade the quality of different pieces of evidence (Carande-Kulis et al., 2000). Other frameworks, such as benefit–cost analysis, have clear criteria for what is to be counted and what is not, but the execution of the analysis must still rely on the analyst's judgment (Nash et al., 1975; Weisbrod, 1983).

A Framework Includes a Method for Weighting and Summarizing

Ultimately, after the users of a framework have listed all the outcomes they value and have measured program outcomes in those terms, they must choose among the programs. That can be hard to do when the valued outcomes take different forms and the strength and weight of evidence supporting them vary across outcomes. Intervention A may provide safer streets and community participation among parents and children; intervention B may provide meals and social interaction for isolated elderly people; interventions C, D, and E may offer still other things of value. Which programs are most valuable? Which should be done if not all can be? Which should be done first?

If there are only a few interventions and only a few outcomes, listing the contributions of each intervention to each outcome can be sufficient to allow people to choose among them. But the more interventions and the more outcomes, the more difficult the choice becomes. In that case people can end up focusing on one outcome, such as health, and ignoring the others, simply because it becomes too difficult to know how to take them all into account. An overall summary measure can help prevent this narrowing of focus, although this is not always possible.

How Do We Know if a Framework Works?

A framework works if it supports an intelligent decision-making process, that is, a process that clarifies trade-offs, reminds decision makers of the things that are important, and helps decision makers explore and work through, rather than gloss over, disagreements. Of course, a particular decision may seem intelligent to one person, while it seems an awful mistake to another. Disagreements on ultimate decisions are inevitable. One sign that a framework works well is if it is perceived as valid and useful by people who disagree vehemently about what decision should be made.

EIGHT EXISTING FRAMEWORKS

The committee has identified eight existing frameworks that have been used to assess the value of community-based preventions:

1. benefit–cost analysis,
2. cost-effectiveness analysis,
3. Congressional Budget Office (CBO) scoring,

4. the PRECEDE–PROCEED framework,
5. the RE-AIM framework,
6. the Health Impact Assessment (HIA) framework,
7. the Community Preventive Services Task Force (CPSTF) guidelines, and
8. the Canadian Health Services Research Foundation (Lomas) Model.

Three of the existing frameworks emerged from the field of economics (benefit–cost analysis, cost-effectiveness analysis, and CBO scoring), while the rest have their roots in the field of public health planning and promotion (PRECEDE–PROCEED, RE-AIM, HIA, CPSTF, and the Lomas model).

The committee's task in analyzing these frameworks is to identify whether they work well for assessing the value of community-based prevention and, if not, why not. The following sections discuss each framework in terms of its decision-making context, its list of valued outcomes, its criteria for admissible evidence, its weights and summarizing, and its limitations.

Benefit–Cost Analysis

Unless otherwise noted, information in the following section was obtained from Carlson et al. (2011) and Weisbrod (1983). The benefit–cost analysis (BCA) framework grew out of the belief that society's problems can be solved systematically through the rigorous application of quantitative scientific principles. BCA was originally developed to guide decisions regarding large-scale government infrastructure projects, such as dam building and flood control projects, and it is geared toward deciding whether a major capital investment is worthwhile (Subcommittee on Evaluation Standards, 1958). (See Box 4-1 for a thorough description of the BCA methodology.)

Decision-Making Context

In the United States BCA has been used mainly by executive branch agencies of the federal government to guide decisions on whether or not to implement infrastructure projects, job training programs, and other social programs. It has also been applied in regulatory impact analyses to decisions such as limits on toxins in drinking water standards.

List of Valued Outcomes

In principle BCA takes a societal perspective, meaning that it takes into account all the things that all the individuals in society care about. This completeness of perspective is BCA's core strength. Ideally the list of valued outcomes includes market-traded goods and services that can be easily expressed in dollars as well as things like fairness and risk avoidance that are either difficult or impossible to express in dollars. In practice analysts find it difficult to document and quantify the value of things like fairness. Generally, a sound BCA will describe the fairness effects in a separate section, sometimes under the label of "intangibles."

Criteria for Admissible Evidence

In general, it is up to the analyst to decide what evidence to include in measuring the quantitative effects of an intervention and the value of those effects. The evidence that is most clearly admissible is high-quality published quantitative evidence on the effect of the policy on some outcome of relevance. Price data for market-traded goods and services that are program outcomes are also admissible. A difficult problem occurs when an important outcome that is affected by the intervention is not traded in markets and, therefore, has no price. In this case, the analyst must rely on systematic reviews of published academic literature on such topics as willingness to pay as well as on expert opinion and on his or her personal judgments. That flexible approach is essential given the comprehensive list of valued outcomes in BCA and the very wide scope of projects to which BCA can be applied. As with some other frameworks for assessing value, this flexibility inevitably requires users to apply judgments regarding the reliability of estimates of benefits and costs.

Weighting and Summarizing

BCA uses a single metric—dollars (or other currency)—to summarize the good and bad effects of an intervention and the resources used to undertake the intervention. Dollar values are assigned in a straightforward way to market-traded goods and services, but they are also assigned to things, such as extended life expectancy that are not traded directly in markets. The concept of "willingness to pay" is used to provide a dollar value for such things as the chance of a better health outcome due to a proposed intervention. All future benefits of a project are summarized in present-value dollars, as are all future costs. The present value of a cost or benefit that occurs in the future is deflated to the present using a discount factor.

The BCA technique uses methods for measuring and describing the degree of uncertainty in the assessment of value. One prominent technique is called Monte Carlo simulation analysis, in which the value of an intervention is assessed repeatedly, each time using assumptions that are drawn randomly (hence "Monte Carlo") from a range of possible values defined

---

BOX 4-1
Benefit–Cost Analysis: Theoretical Basis
and Practical Considerations

Benefit–cost analysts seek to identify both private and public decisions in which the benefits (or outputs) are greater than the costs (or inputs).

Market prices should be used to measure the value of both benefits and costs, except where market prices do not exist or when there is a good reason to believe that market prices do not accurately reflect true value. Among the reasons for questioning the appropriateness of observed prices are the existence of monopoly power in particular sectors, economies of scale, a serious lack of information, or external effects (or spillovers) not reflected in market values.

Where the prices of inputs or outputs do not exist, analysts strive to construct values that reflect people's valuation of inputs and outcomes. (These are known as *shadow values* or *shadow prices*.)

Although economic efficiency should be regarded as the primary objective, when decisions have important equity (and other) effects, these should be recorded and, if possible, entered into the benefit–cost analysis itself. An alternative way of describing the efficiency criterion is to state that projects should be designed to maximize total (or per capita) national economic welfare, which is often assumed to be equivalent to national income. To do this the project should maximize the net benefits that it generates.

Benefits (or costs) that will not occur until sometime into the future should be valued (weighted) as less important (per dollar) than benefits or costs expected to be incurred immediately because (and only if) this reflects how people feel about future benefits and costs relative to present ones. The process employed for making benefits and costs which occur at different points in time commensurable is called discounting and requires the use of a discount (or interest) rate to reflect the diminished value today of benefits or costs not expected to occur until some future time period. For projects that generate a stream of future benefits or costs, the benefit–cost ratio (B/C) is

B/C = Total discounted value of future expected benefits/
Total discounted value of future expected costs, or

Net Present Value of Program = Present value of benefits/
Present value of costs

---

by the analyst. This enables the user to see the range of possible outcomes under various combinations of assumptions as well as the likelihood that they will be realized (Savvides, 1994).

More Details and Examples

Among the many published BCA studies, two of the most comprehensive are Weisbrod's (1983) analysis of non-institutional care for the

An intervention has externality, or spillover, effects if it affects individuals who do not directly participate. Externalities, which can be positive or negative, should be accounted for in a benefit–cost analysis, even if observed market prices are not available for the valuation of the effect.

The concept of "benefit" (which when negative becomes a "cost") underlies all benefit–cost analyses; a clear understanding of the meaning of "benefit" is the fundamental requirement for undertaking any sound benefit–cost study of public activities. It is useful to think of the benefits of a public intervention as the extent to which the program produces desirable results. What is or is not desirable depends, in turn, on the goals or objectives of the program. This is to say, the first step in the process of project evaluation or policy analysis should be a statement of goals. The second step should be an attempt to state these goals in operationally measurable form. The third step in the analysis is the development of a set of weights that reflect judgments about the comparative importance of progress toward each of the goals—the goal trade-offs.

Valued outcomes in BCA can be grouped into two principal categories: (1) those related to economic allocative efficiency and (2) those related to distributional equity.

Allocative efficiency as an economic goal reflects the fact that it is sometimes possible to reallocate resources—perhaps increasing or decreasing the amount of resources used in any expenditure program in ways that will bring about an increase in the net value of output produced by those resources. For such reallocations the increase in the value of the output of the good whose production is expanded must be greater than the decrease in the value of the output of the good whose production is decreased. Insofar as benefit–cost analysis is directed at allocative efficiency, it can be viewed as an attempt to replicate for the public sector the decisions that would be made if private markets worked satisfactorily (Haveman and Weisbrod, 1977). However, allocative efficiency ignores considerations of which particular people are made better off or worse off. The issue of how alternative resource allocations affect the well-being of particular people is captured by the distributional—or equity—goals. The goals can and should be incorporated into benefit–cost analysis, but must be done explicitly. One way of examining distributional effects is through sensitivity analysis, which varies the values of certain inputs to determine their influence on output.

mentally ill and Carlson et al.'s (2011) analysis of Section 8 housing subsidies.

Shortcomings of BCA When Applied to Assessing the Value of Community-Based Prevention

BCA requires a monetary assessment of how a community trades one outcome for another. However, some outcomes, such as social cohesion or civic participation are not readily monetized, and there are other factors, such as years of human life, that can (and have been monetized), but for which monetization is controversial. An example of the latter can be seen in the value of a year of human life assigned in the regulatory impact analyses conducted by the Environmental Protection Agency (IOM, 2006).

Cost-Effectiveness Analysis

Cost-effectiveness analysis (CEA) begins with many of the core elements of BCA framework, but it is tailored to the assessment of medical and health interventions. The key difference between CEA and BCA is that CEA focuses on health as the valued outcome and measures health by methods that avoid the use of dollars (Donaldson, 1998; Gold et al., 1996). The measures of health often used in CEA include cases of disease, life-years, and health-adjusted life expectancy. The core question that CEA answers is how much it costs to produce an additional unit of health using one particular intervention versus a second intervention with which it is compared (Bleichrodt and Quiggin, 1999; Donaldson, 1998; Drummond et al., 2005; Gold et al., 1996).

The answer to this question is given by what is termed the "cost-effectiveness ratio." An intervention's cost-effectiveness ratio is, in effect, the dollars spent for an additional unit of health. The health measure that is the standard of good practice is quality-adjusted life years (QALYs), so that the cost-effectiveness of an intervention is thus expressed as the additional cost to achieve an additional QALY (Gold et al., 1996). A cost-effectiveness ratio, sometimes called an incremental cost-effectiveness ratio, is not a fixed or single number associated with an intervention. It is instead defined with reference to some alternative intervention, and thus its value depends on what the alternative is. For example, vaccinating children once in early childhood may be compared with not vaccinating them but instead treating the disease when it occurs. Or providing a single vaccination could be compared with providing multiple vaccinations over time, perhaps including a booster in adulthood. The cost-effectiveness of vaccinating once will differ depending on which comparison is chosen.

Decision-Making Context

CEA is geared toward maximizing the health improvements achieved among a target population and to analyzing the resources or costs likely to be required to achieve those health improvements. An example of this sort of decision-making context is provided by the Department of Veterans Affairs, which operates a health system on a fixed budget with the goal of improving the health of its enrolled population. CEA can help the administrator of that program prioritize technology adoption and choose the treatment guidelines that produce health improvements most efficiently. Cost-effectiveness analysis is not used explicitly in the development of coverage policy and practice guidelines in the United States.

In other countries cost-effectiveness is often explicitly used to help set standards of care and coverage. The UK National Institute for Health and Clinical Excellence (NICE) uses cost-effectiveness analysis as one element in deciding whether the National Health Service (NHS) will pay for new technologies; its purpose is to help ensure that everyone in the country has access to proven medical care (Steinbrook, 2008). NICE sometimes uses cost-effectiveness analysis to negotiate prices with manufacturers who can improve the cost-effectiveness of their product by reducing its price (Kanis et al., 2008; Steinbrook, 2008). Australia's Pharmaceutical Benefits Advisory Committee (PBAC) uses cost-effectiveness analysis to develop guidance for the Minister of Health on the medications that should be covered by the national pharmacy benefits plan (Department of Health and Aging, 2007; Henry et al., 2005).

List of Valued Outcomes

Health is the primary valued outcome in CEA. CEA takes into account the health improvements and adverse effects from the intervention that occur over a specific time horizon, often the lifetime of patients, to calculate the net health benefits, which are defined as improvements minus adverse effects. As noted, health improvements include both longer life and better quality of life. CEA calculates the resources used to produce the health improvements separately. Resources include market-traded items, such as physician labor, hospital care, and pharmaceuticals, as well as non-market-traded items, such as patients' time and the time of unpaid caregivers. The health improvements and costs of an intervention are then compared with an alternative intervention—vaccination with waiting and treating illness, screening annually with screening less often, and so on—in order to arrive at the net addition to health and the net addition to costs (or savings) of the intervention compared to the alternative. The cost-effectiveness ratio is the net costs divided by the net addition to health (Gold et al., 1996; Weinstein and Stason, 1977).

Criteria for Admissible Evidence

In general the modeling team uses the best available evidence, with preference given to published peer-reviewed literature (Gold et al., 1996). When published data are not available, the team is expected to use judgment and expert opinion to fill in key parameters when published data are not available. In the United States the standards for admissible evidence have moved rapidly in the direction of requiring systematic reviews of the literature, published and unpublished (Harris et al., 2001; U.S. Preventive Services Task Force, 2012). If many studies are available in the literature, a meta-analysis is used to summarize them and arrive at the best estimate of the effectiveness of an intervention. The move toward systematic reviews has followed the trend in other countries set by the Cochrane Collaboration, headquartered in the United Kingdom. The Cochrane Collaboration draws on experts in more than 100 countries to prepare and make available on its website systematic reviews of the medical, public health, and related applied sciences literature on thousands of health topics (Cochrane Collaboration, 2012). The standards it has developed for such reviews are increasingly used around the world.

Weighting and Summarizing

Changes in health status are usually summarized using QALYs, which reflect both length of a life and its quality (e.g., a year of perfect health counts as 1.0 QALY, while years of less-than-perfect health are given scores between 0 and 1 depending on the severity of illness [Gold et al., 1996]). The health effects of an intervention are given by the sum of all the changes in QALYs, good and bad, compared to an alternative intervention. Here, as with BCA, sensitivity analysis can be instructive as to distributional aspects of the proposed intervention. It can be difficult, however, to build equity considerations into the analysis (IOM, 2006). Future changes are discounted so that QALYs are expressed in present value. Resource use— that is, costs—is also summarized in discounted (present-value) dollars. The incremental cost-effectiveness ratio (ICER) compares the discounted QALYs and costs of the intervention with those of alternative interventions, as described, and might be thought of as a price tag to use to prioritize interventions: How much would it cost to produce one healthy year using this intervention rather than the one with which it is compared?

More Details and Examples

Hundreds of CEAs are published each year by medical and health journals and by advisory groups such as NICE and the Australian PBAC. The authoritative description of CEA methodology is by Gold et al. (1996); Appendixes B and C of that report describe two examples of CEA—the cost-effectiveness of interventions to prevent neural tube defects (Appendix B) and the cost-effectiveness of interventions to reduce cholesterol in adults (Appendix C).

Shortcomings of CEA When Applied to Assessing the Value of Community-Based Prevention

The primary shortcoming of CEA as a method for valuing community-based prevention is that it focuses solely on the aggregation of individual health outcomes. It does not include—and has not developed methodologies to measure—the effects of an intervention on community well-being or community process and does not usually take into consideration the differences among communities (Birch and Gafni, 2003).

Congressional Budget Office Scoring

The Congressional Budget Office (CBO) is a nonpartisan congressional support agency that analyzes existing federal programs and proposed legislation to provide budget, economic, and other information for Congress. The agency staff is made up of economists and research staff who develop cost estimates, reports, and other products. Cost estimates, often called CBO "scores," are projections of the federal budget impact of a piece of legislation being considered by the Congress.

Some of the legislation that CBO scores relates to prevention. Often the scores have been criticized for failing to fully recognize the benefits of prevention (Woolf et al., 2009). But CBO's framework for assessing value is designed to aid in the federal budget process—it is not designed to provide a comprehensive assessment of the value of prevention activities. It is, therefore, unsurprising that advocates for prevention activities feel ill-served by CBO's assessments.

Decision-Making Context

CBO scores play a formal role in the federal budget process. Because the scores are designed to help the House and Senate budget committees ensure that legislation fits within a larger budget framework, CBO details the *budget* impact of proposed policies. A consistent framework for presenting information—defined in law[1] and through formal agreements between the House and Senate budget committees—helps lawmakers consider the absolute and relative budget costs of different policies and programs, from health to income security and defense.

---

[1] Budget Enforcement Act of 1990. Public Law 508, 101st Cong., 1st sess. (November 5, 1990).

List of Valued Outcomes

CBO scoring emphasizes one outcome: changes in the federal deficit over the next 10 years. To measure that outcome, cost estimates detail projected changes in federal revenues and federal outlays. Written cost estimates sometimes include information about health impact and other outcomes of interest (for example, expected changes in smoking rates from amendments to the Food, Drug, and Cosmetic Act or expected changes in insurance coverage under the Affordable Care Act), but discussion of these non-budget outcomes is limited. CBO scores must also include a statement indicating whether proposed legislation would impose an "unfunded mandate" on either the private sector or on state and local governments.

Criteria for Admissible Evidence

In general, modelers at CBO use the best available evidence, including published academic literature, expert opinion, and the modeler's judgment (Kling, 2011). CBO cannot decline to produce an estimate due to lack of evidence, so casting a broad net for evidence is essential.

Weighting and Summarizing

The primary measure for CBO scoring—the estimated 10-year change in the federal deficit—is presented in total and is also broken down to detail various submeasures, which include changes in revenues, changes in outlays, annual changes in revenues and outlays, changes in outlays for mandatory programs (such as Medicare), and changes in outlays for discretionary programs (such as CDC). Details about the submeasures fulfill the needs of the federal budget process, where revenue, spending, and other budget categories must be tracked separately.

More Details and Examples

For an example of a cost estimate of health-related legislation, see CBO's scoring of the Family Smoking Prevention and Tobacco Control Act (2008). For a general discussion of CBO's use of evidence and approach to scoring, see Kling (2011).

Shortcomings of CBO Scoring When Applied to Assessing the Value of Community-Based Prevention

The most obvious shortcoming of CBO's framework is its focus, as required by legislation, on changes in the federal deficit. By design, CBO's framework does not emphasize the inherent value of health improvements or other improvements in well-being from community-based prevention. Policy makers can and do take such non-budget factors into account when making decisions, even when not addressed in CBO analyses.

Another shortcoming is the use of the 10-year budget window, which can be too short to pick up some important outcomes, such as long-term health improvements from policies or programs that reduce childhood obesity. Finally, the process of selecting policies for scoring is very limited— formal cost estimates are produced only for pieces of legislation that have been reported out of a committee of Congress.

The PRECEDE–PROCEED Framework

As noted in Chapter 2, the PRECEDE–PROCEED model is a widely applied framework for decision making in the planning and evaluation of health-promotion and disease-prevention programs and services. The ecological approach of that framework has particular relevance to community- or population-level efforts (Green and Kreuter, 2005). PRECEDE is an acronym for predisposing, reinforcing, and enabling constructs in educational/ecological diagnosis and evaluation, while PROCEED similarly refers to other anchors in the model: policy, regulatory, and organizational constructs in educational and ecological development. The combination of these elements in planning and evaluation constitute a framework both as a logic model and as a procedural model.

Decision-Making Context

This model is used extensively in courses on planning and evaluation in schools of public health and other graduate programs in the health sciences. It is widely applied by program planners, community health advisory boards, and practitioners. Among those applications more than 1,000 have been published (Green, 2012c).

List of Valued Outcomes

In general, the valued outcomes include health and quality of life, but the outcomes used to evaluate a specific program will depend on the program's goals or, among those, the specific objectives that the community planners select for evaluation. Quality of life can encompass a broad array of community-level indicators of well-being. The framework puts heavy emphasis on the process of developing and carrying out a health promotion process of planning, and the inclusion of community members and stakeholders in the development of a program is a valued outcome in and of itself (Harvey and O'Brien, 2011; Watson et al., 2001).

Criteria for Admissible Evidence

PRECEDE–PROCEED emphasizes the blending of evidence matched with each of several ecological levels, with theory applicable to each of those levels, with professional experience, and with community perspectives derived from a participatory process of planning and research (Green and Kreuter, 2005).

Weighting and Summarizing

The PRECEDE–PROCEED approach is not designed to produce a weighted summary measure of the expected impact of an intervention, but it does include procedures for the valuing process of considering the relative importance attached to each intended outcome from the professionals' and public's perspectives.

More Details and Examples

Many of the more than 1,000 published applications, tests, reviews, and reflections relating to PRECEDE–PROCEED have focused on developing, valuing, or evaluating interventions, programs, and policies in specific community settings, such as school health promotion or worksite wellness programs, or have examined specific components such as the mass media component of a program or the policy impact of a new law or regulation (Buta et al., 2011; Green, 2012a). Some are adaptations of more comprehensive applications of previously tested or mandated programs for mass immunization or screening, which makes them community-*placed* programs. The full application of the model produces a community-*based* program as it engages the community more actively in setting priorities and blending components of the policies, programs, settings, strategies, and tactics to be included and monitored.

Shortcomings of PRECEDE–PROCEED When Applied to Prospective Valuing of Community-Based Prevention

The participatory orientation of PRECEDE–PROCEED is its strength, but it also limits its usefulness for a funding agency wanting to assess the value of many different possible interventions. In the PRECEDE–PROCEED framework the value of an intervention—and the nature of the intervention itself—depends on local conditions and the input and guidance of the community. This framework does not assess the resources used to conduct an intervention, and so cannot be used to weigh costs against benefits.

The Reach, Effectiveness, Adoption, Implementation, and Maintenance (RE-AIM) Framework

Decision-Making Context

The RE-AIM framework has been widely used in the community health promotion field to assess whether a specific intervention is likely to have a positive impact on health (Glasgow et al., 1999).

List of Valued Outcomes

The only valued outcome in the RE-AIM framework is an improvement in population health, although that outcome will be specified differently depending on the intervention. RE-AIM measures resource use as an outcome.

Criteria for Admissible Evidence

In general the modeler uses the best available evidence, including expert opinion and the modeler's judgment.

Weighting and Summarizing

An intervention is summarized on five dimensions: reach (the share of the population reached by the intervention), effectiveness (of those reached, the share who get a positive result), adoption (the share of the population served by organizations that adopt the program), implementation (the share of adopting organizations that implement the program), and maintenance (the share of implementing organizations that maintain the program). These five elements of a program or intervention can be seen as multiplicative, insofar as each depends for its impact on health on the level of the others (Glasgow et al., 1999). Thus, if each has a yield of 0.5 for a particular program, the result will be $.5 \times .5 \times .5 \times .5 \times .5 = 3.1$ percent of the eligible population getting a positive result.

More Details and Examples

The website http://www.RE-AIM.org offers a growing list of publications that have tested the RE-AIM components or applied RE-AIM in the prospective valuing and retrospective evaluation of programs (NCI, 2012). It is sometimes combined with PRECEDE–PROCEED and other planning models in health promotion and clinical programs. One application of RE-AIM that is particularly relevant to valuing interventions for programs is its use in the development of guidelines for assessing the external validity, or generalizability, of the results of experimental and other evaluation results (Green and Glasgow, 2006; Green et al., 2009). This set of guidelines developed with the use of RE-AIM has been adopted or recommended by several journals as guidelines for authors (Green, 2012b).

Shortcomings of RE-AIM When Applied to Assessing the Value of Community-Based Prevention

RE-AIM does not specify individual or community-level health measures except insofar as they are used as the measure of "effectiveness." Ideally, calculations of effectiveness in RE-AIM rely on health measures, but they sometimes use health risk behaviors or changes in community health risk conditions (Glasgow et al., 1999).

Health Impact Assessment

The Health Impact Assessment (HIA) is a framework for assessing the health impacts of interventions primarily in non-health sectors for the purpose of mitigating potential harms or enhancing potential benefits. HIAs can be used to examine policies, such as living wage laws, zoning restrictions to reduce sensitive use development around high-use roadways, or agricultural subsidies as well as to assess projects, such as the development of a subway system or the introduction of a farmer's market. HIAs are used as a way to introduce health considerations into all policies (i.e, "health in all policies" or HiAP) (IOM, 2011). The steps in conducting an HIA are shown in Figure 4-1.

Decision-Making Context

HIAs are used to provide decision makers, usually in non-health sectors, with information on the health effects of policies and projects. In addition they provide information about how to modify policies or projects so that health impacts can be improved, i.e., the harms reduced or the benefits enhanced. The HIA has been more widely used in Europe than in the United States, but its use has increased in the last 10 years, and the approach has gained increased visibility through capacity building supported by the Pew Charitable Trusts and the Robert Wood Johnson Foundation (Pew Charitable Trusts, 2009; RWJF, 2009). A recent report, *Improving Health in the United States* (NRC, 2011) provided guidance to provide more standardization for HIAs.

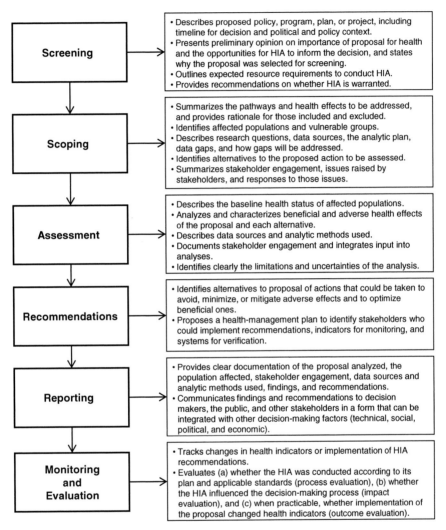

FIGURE 4-1 Framework for a Health Impact Assessment, illustrating steps and outputs.
SOURCE: NRC, 2011.

List of Valued Outcomes

HIAs do not have a specific list of health outcomes to evaluate. Rather, a scoping process, including literature reviews and expert consultation, is used to identify the potential health impacts that are of importance to the affected stakeholders. The level of stakeholder participation varies with the type of policy or project. For example, the development of new residential and commercial infrastructure would engage those currently living in the area as well as individuals in the business and other communities. Considerations might include the effects of displacement, the disruption of social networks and cohesion, increased housing cost, changes in access to public transportation, and changes in job prospects as well as the impact of commercial development (London's Health, 2000; UCLA HIA-CLIC, 2012).

Criteria for Admissible Evidence

In general the best available information is used to assess the health impact. Evidence may be qualitative or quantitative. The degree of rigor is often contingent on the nature of the project, the analytic resources available, the urgency of the decision makers, and the time available (Snowdon et al., 2010).

Weighting and Summarizing

Changes in health status are usually displayed in natural health units and are sometimes summarized using QALYs.

More Details and Examples

The 2011 NRC report *Improving Health in the United States* provides a summary of the purposes, methods, and uses of HIAs.

Shortcomings of HIA When Applied to Assessing the Value of Community-Based Prevention

The primary shortcoming of HIA is that it does not capture the costs associated with an intervention. Analyses are adapted to the specific interventions and stakeholders and thus they can vary significantly (Kemm, 2003).

Community Preventive Services Task Force Guidelines

The Community Preventive Services Task Force (CPSTF) is an independent, nonfederal, volunteer body with members appointed by the Director of the Centers for Disease Control and Prevention (CDC). Those members represent a broad range of research, practice, and policy expertise in community preventive services, public health, health promotion, and disease prevention (Community Guide, 2012d). See Box 4-2 for CPSTF Prioritization Process.

Decision-Making Context

The CPSTF recommendations influence decisions of the CDC and of other funders regarding which activities to fund. Local health departments, community groups, and health systems also use the recommendations to decide which interventions to undertake (Community Guide, 2012b).

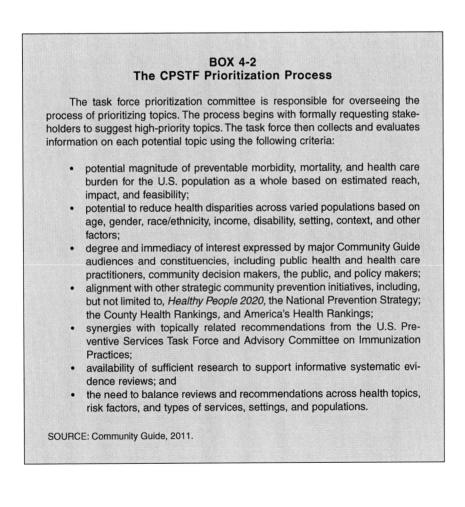

BOX 4-2
The CPSTF Prioritization Process

The task force prioritization committee is responsible for overseeing the process of prioritizing topics. The process begins with formally requesting stakeholders to suggest high-priority topics. The task force then collects and evaluates information on each potential topic using the following criteria:

- potential magnitude of preventable morbidity, mortality, and health care burden for the U.S. population as a whole based on estimated reach, impact, and feasibility;
- potential to reduce health disparities across varied populations based on age, gender, race/ethnicity, income, disability, setting, context, and other factors;
- degree and immediacy of interest expressed by major Community Guide audiences and constituencies, including public health and health care practitioners, community decision makers, the public, and policy makers;
- alignment with other strategic community prevention initiatives, including, but not limited to, *Healthy People 2020*, the National Prevention Strategy; the County Health Rankings, and America's Health Rankings;
- synergies with topically related recommendations from the U.S. Preventive Services Task Force and Advisory Committee on Immunization Practices;
- availability of sufficient research to support informative systematic evidence reviews; and
- the need to balance reviews and recommendations across health topics, risk factors, and types of services, settings, and populations.

SOURCE: Community Guide, 2011.

List of Valued Outcomes

The CPSTF evaluates the effectiveness of interventions (programs and policies). The key valued outcome is the health of a population, assessed as the sum of the health of individuals. The CPSTF guidelines also measures how effective interventions are in different populations (distributional and equity effects), generalizability, and acceptability (Community Guide, 2012c). For those interventions where there is evidence of effectiveness the resource use and cost-effectiveness are assessed where studies are available, although these are not used for making the primary recommendation (Hahn et al., 2004).

Criteria for Admissible Evidence

The CPSTF guidelines are based on systematic reviews of the published academic literature. The admissibility of published studies is determined according to the appropriateness of the study design for the intervention being examined and the quality of execution. The criteria recognize that randomized controlled trials may not be the most appropriate study design and that they are often impractical for assessment of community-level interventions. Thus, well-done observational studies are often included (Norris et al., 2002).

Weighting and Summarizing

The findings from the literature review are summarized on two dimensions: Is the evidence strong enough to draw a conclusion (i.e., are there enough studies of suitable design and execution)? And, if so, does the evidence indicate that the intervention improves health outcomes? (The Community Guide, 2012a).

More Details and Examples

For a detailed description of CPSTF's methodology see Briss et al. (2000) and Carande-Kulis et al. (2000). The CPSTF's recommendations are available at http://www.thecommunityguide.org/index.html.

Shortcomings of the CPSTF Guidelines When Applied to Assessing the Value of Community-Based Prevention

The CPSTF guidelines have several shortcomings: The list of valued outcomes focuses only on outcomes associated with health; the process for determining which interventions are studied is highly centralized; and conclusions do not consider the tradeoff between benefits and costs, although where cost effectiveness information is available that information is summarized.

The Canadian Health Services Research Foundation Model

The Canadian Health Services Research Foundation (CHSRF) model—also referred to as the Lomas model after Jonathan Lomas, the first chief executive officer of the CHSRF—provides a conceptual framework for combining evidence of different types to inform health system decision making. It is not a full-fledged framework for assessing value because it does not specify a list of valued outcomes. Instead, it enumerates the different types of evidence used by different decision makers (Lomas et al., 2005).

Decision-Making Context

The model focuses on the use of evidence in real-world decision making and recognizes that a broad range of information, correct or incorrect, is used by decision makers. The primary focus is on how those who formulate guidance use different types of evidence in making their recommendations, setting their targets, and providing guidance (Lomas et al., 2005).

List of Valued Outcomes

The Lomas model does not specify a set of valued outcomes.

Criteria for Admissible Evidence

The model describes different types of evidence, but it does not have specific criteria for what may be included. All types of evidence are, in general, admissible, which is the generally accepted practice of the relevant disciplines and decision makers.

The Lomas model distinguishes three types of evidence: scientific evidence, social science scientific evidence, and colloquial evidence. Scientific evidence is considered context-independent—that is, the information is knowable and broadly true. It provides information about whether an intervention *can* work. The efficacy result of a randomized controlled trial is a typical example. Social science scientific evidence is considered to be context dependent—that is, the information is knowable, but the result depends on the context in which it occurs. Such evidence provides information about whether an intervention *does* work in a given community. Effectiveness studies are an example. The final type of evidence, colloquial evidence, "can usefully be divided into evidence about resources, expert and professional opinion, political judgment, values, habits and traditions, lob-byists and pressure groups, and the particular pragmatics and contingencies of the situation" (Lomas et al., 2005, p. 1).

Weighting and Summarizing

The Lomas model does not prescribe a single approach for weight-ing or summarizing the various pieces of evidence, and it recognizes the importance of all types of evidence and the lack of a technical solution to making the best choice. This framework incorporates a deliberative process of relevant stakeholders to consider and weigh all the different types of information.

More Details and Examples

See Lomas et al. (2005).

Shortcomings of the Lomas Model When Applied to Assessing the Value of Community-Based Prevention

The Lomas model does not specify a list of valued outcomes or a method for weighting and summarizing an intervention's impacts. The Lomas model is more descriptive of the decision-making process and is not meant to be prescriptive or normative (Lomas et al., 2005).

VALUING COMMUNITY-BASED PREVENTION: IS A NEW FRAMEWORK NEEDED?

This chapter has identified eight existing frameworks for assessing value. Given the profusion of frameworks, is it really necessary to define another one? The answer depends on how well each of the eight frame-works addresses the special characteristics of community-based prevention described in Chapters 2 and 3.

The committee concluded that a framework for evaluating community preventive programs and policies should meet at least three criteria:

1. The framework should account for benefits and harms in three domains: health, community well-being, and community process (see Chapter 3). Community-based prevention can create value not only through improvements in the health of individuals but also by increasing the investment individuals are willing and able

to make in themselves, in their family and neighbors, and in their environment. Furthermore, community-based prevention, by definition, involves decisions among groups of people about how to live in society, how the physical environment should be built, what food should be served in schools, and so on. Thus, the process by which interventions are decided upon and undertaken needs to be treated as a valued outcome. If a community decides to tell people what they can or cannot do or what they should or should not do, the decisions need to have the legitimacy—the added value—that comes from an open and inclusive group decision-making process.

2. The framework should consider the resources used and compare benefits and harms with those resources. To make that comparison, and to compare different interventions with each other, it is essential not only to know that some benefit is likely, but also to be aware of the magnitude of the benefits and of the costs associated with each intervention.

3. The framework needs to be sensitive to differences among communities and to take them into account in valuing community-based prevention. In part this reflects the reality that, because communities vary so much in their characteristics, the causal links between interventions and valued outcomes may be different for different communities.

None of the eight frameworks meets all three criteria—that is, accounts for benefits and harms in all three domains identified in Chapter 3, compares benefits with costs, and is sensitive to differences among communities (see Table 4-1). Only three of the eight are comprehensive in accounting for benefits and can thus assess value in all three domains of health, community well-being, and community process. Only three estimate costs as a matter of course. Four are moderate or high in their attention to differences among communities. Benefit–cost analysis, which is comprehensive in accounting for benefits and always estimates costs, does not routinely consider the unique characteristics of the decision-making context and the community. PRECEDE–PROCEED, which measures health and community process benefits and takes the unique characteristics of the community into account, does not require that costs be estimated.

The committee concluded that a new framework is necessary to guide the assessment of value for community-based prevention, one that measures benefits comprehensively, compares benefits with costs, and takes into account the differences among and within communities. Chapter 5 describes such a new framework.

TABLE 4-1   Eight Frameworks Summarized

	Includes Comprehensive Set of Valued Outcomes	Compares Benefits with Costs	Accounts for Differences Among Communities
Benefit–cost analysis (BCA)	Yes, can account for all benefits	Yes	Low; can account for context
Cost-effectiveness analysis	No, health only	Yes	Low; can account for context
Congressional Budget Office scoring	No, only federal spending and revenue	Yes	Low; designed for Congressional budget process
PRECEDE–PROCEED framework	No, although it includes both health and community process	No	High; used in communities
RE-AIM framework	No, health only	No	High; used by evaluators
Health Impact Assessment framework	No, health only	No	High; used in communities
Community Preventive Services Task Force guidelines	No, health only	No	Moderate; focus on community
Lomas model	No, valued outcomes not specified	No	Moderate; focus on decision-making process

REFERENCES

Birch, S., and A. Gafni. 2003. Economics and the evaluation of health care programmes: Generalisability of methods and implications for generalisability of results. *Health Policy* 64(2):207-219.

Bleichrodt, H., and J. Quiggin. 1999. Life-cycle preferences over consumption and health: When is cost-effectiveness analysis equivalent to cost–benefit analysis? *Journal of Health Economics* 18(6):681-708.

Briss, P. A., S. Zaza, M. Pappaioanou, J. Fielding, L. Wright-De Agüero, B. I. Truman, D. P. Hopkins, P. D. Mullen, R. S. Thompson, and S. H. Woolf. 2000. Developing an evidence-based guide to community preventive services: Methods. The Task Force on Community Preventive Services. *American Journal of Preventive Medicine* 18(1 Suppl):35-43.

Buta, B., L. Brewer, D. L. Hamlin, M. W. Palmer, J. Bowie, and A. Gielen. 2011. An innovative faith-based healthy eating program: From class assignment to real-world application of PRECEDE–PROCEED. *Health Promotion Practice* 12(6):867-875.

Carande-Kulis, V. G., M. V. Maciosek, P. A. Briss, S. M. Teutsch, S. Zaza, B. I. Truman, M. L. Messonnier, M. Pappaioanou, J. R. Harris, and J. Fielding. 2000. Methods for systematic reviews of economic evaluations for the Guide to Community Preventive Services. *American Journal of Preventive Medicine* 18:75-91.

Carlson, D., R. Haveman, T. Kaplan, and B. Wolfe. 2011. The benefits and costs of the Section 8 housing subsidy program: A framework and estimates of first year effects. *Journal of Policy Analysis and Management* 30(2):233-255.

CBO (Congressional Budget Office). 2008. *Family Smoking Prevention and Tobacco Control Act.* Washington, DC: Congressional Budget Office.

Cochrane Collaboration. 2012. *About us: The Cochrance Collaboration.* http://www.cochrane.org/about-us (accessed May 21, 2012).

Community Guide. 2011. *Community Preventive Services Task Force first annual report to Congress.* Atlanta, GA: Community Preventive Services Task Force.

Community Guide. 2012a. *The Community Guide—systematic review methods.* http://www.thecommunityguide.org/about/methods.html (accessed May 22, 2012).

Community Guide. 2012b. *The Community Preventive Services Task Force.* http://www.thecommunityguide.org/about/task-force-members.html (accessed May 22, 2012).

Community Guide. 2012c. *The guide to community preventive services.* http://www.thecommunityguide.org/index.html (accessed May 22, 2012).

Community Guide. 2012d. *What is the Community Preventive Services Task Force?* http://www.thecommunityguide.org/about/aboutTF.html (accessed May 22, 2012).

Department of Health and Aging. 2007. *Pharmaceutical Benefits Advisory Committee.* http://www.health.gov.au/internet/main/publishing.nsf/content/health-pbs-general-listing-committee3.htm (accessed May 21, 2012).

Donaldson, C. 1998. The (near) equivalence of cost-effectiveness and cost-benefit analyses: Fact or fallacy? *Pharmacoeconomics* 13(4):389-396.

Drummond, M., M. Schulper, G. Torrance, B. Obrien, and G. Stoddart. 2005. *Methods for economic evaluation of health care programmes.* 3rd Ed. New York: Oxford University Press Inc.

Glasgow, R. E., T. M. Vogt, and S. M. Boles. 1999. Evaluating the public health impact of health promotion interventions: The RE-AIM framework. *American Journal of Public Health* 89(9):1322-1327.

Gold, M., J. Siegel, L. Russell, and M. Weinstein. 1996. *Cost-effectiveness in health and medicine.* New York: Oxford University Press.

Green, L. W. 2012a. *Bibliographies.* http://lgreen.net/bibliog.htm (accessed May 22, 2012).

Green, L. W. 2012b. Furthering dissemination and implementation research: The need for more attention to eternal validity. In *Dissemination and implementation research in health: Translating science to practice,* edited by R. C. Brownson, G. A. Colditz, and E. K. Proctor. New York: Oxford University Press. Pp. 305-326.

Green, L. W. 2012c. *PRECEDE applications.* http://lgreen.net/precede%20apps/preapps-NEW.htm (accessed May 22, 2012).

Green, L. W., and R. E. Glasgow. 2006. Evaluating the relevance, generalization, and applicability of research. *Evaluation and the Health Professions* 29(1):126-153.

Green, L. W., and M. W. Kreuter. 2005. *Health program planning: an educational and ecological approach,* 4th ed. New York: McGraw-Hill.

Green, L. W., R. E. Glasgow, D. Atkins, and K. Stange. 2009. Making evidence from research more relevant, useful, and actionable in policy, program planning, and practice: Slips "twixt cup and lip". *American Journal of Preventive Medicine* 37(6):S187-S191.

Hahn, R. A., J. Lowy, O. Bilukha, S. Snyder, P. Briss, A. Crosby, and P. Corso. 2004. Therapeutic foster care for the prevention of violence. *Morbidity and Mortality Weekly Report* 53(RR10):1-8.

Harris, R. P., M. Helfand, S. H. Woolf, K. N. Lohr, C. D. Mulrow, S. M. Teutsch, and D. Atkins. 2001. Current methods of the U.S. Preventive Services Task Force: A review of the process. *American Journal of Preventive Medicine* 20(3 Suppl):21-35.

Harvey, I., and M. O'Brien. 2011. Addressing health disparities through patient education: The development of culturally tailored health education materials at Puentes de Salud. *Journal of Community Health Nursing* 28(4):181-189.

Haveman, R., and B. A. Weisbrod. 1977. Public expenditure and policy analysis: An overview. In *Public expenditure and policy analysis*, edited by R. Haveman and J. Margolis. Skokie, IL: Rand McNally College. Pp. 1-24.

Henry, D. A., S. R. Hill, and A. Harris. 2005. Drug prices and value for money. *JAMA* 294(20):2630-2632.

IOM (Institute of Medicine). 2006. *Valuing health for regulatory cost-effectiveness analysis.* Washington, DC: The National Academies Press.

IOM. 2011. *For the public's health: Revitalizing law and policy to meet new challenges.* Washington, DC: The National Academies Press.

Kanis, J. A., J. Adams, F. Borgström, C. Cooper, B. Jönsson, D. Preedy, P. Selby, and J. Compston. 2008. The cost-effectiveness of alendronate in the management of osteoporosis. *Bone* 42(1):4-15.

Kemm, J. 2003. Perspectives on health impact assessment. *Bulletin of the World Health Organization* 81(6):387-387.

Kling, J. R. 2011. *CBO's use of evidence in analysis of budget and economic policies.* http:// www.cbo.gov/sites/default/files/cbofiles/attachments/11-03-APPAM-Presentation_0.pdf (accessed May 21, 2012).

Lomas, J., T. Culyer, C. McCutcheon, L. McAuley, and S. Law. 2005. *Conceptualizing and combining evidence for health system guidance.* Ottawa, Ontario: Canadian Health Services Research Foundation.

London's Health. 2000. *A short guide to health impact assessment: Informing healthy decisions.* London: NHS Executive London.

Nash, C., D. Pearce, and J. Stanley. 1975. An evaluation of cost-benefit analysis criteria. *Scottish Journal of Political Economy* 22(2):121-134.

NCI (National Cancer Institute). 2012. *RE-AIM publications.* http://publications.cancer.gov/ dipubs/reaim.aspx (accessed May 22, 2012).

Norris, S. L., P. J. Nichols, C. J. Caspersen, R. E. Glasgow, M. M. Engelgau, L. Jack, S. R. Snyder, V. G. Carande-Kulis, G. Isham, and S. Garfield. 2002. Increasing diabetes self-management education in community settings: A systematic review. *American Journal of Preventive Medicine* 22(4):39-66.

NRC (National Research Council). 2011. *Improving health in the United States: The role of health impact assessment.* Washington, DC: The National Academies Press.

Pew Charitable Trusts. 2009. *Overview: Health impact project.* http://www.pewtrusts.org/ news_room_detail.aspx?id=55601 (accessed May 22, 2012).

RWJF (Robert Wood Johnson Foundation). 2009. *RWJF, the Pew Charitable Trusts launch health impact project.* http://www.rwjf.org/publichealth/product.jsp?id=50088 (accessed May 22, 2012).

Savvides, S. 1994. Risk analysis in investment appraisal. *Project Appraisal Journal* 9(1):3-18.

Snowdon, W., J.-L. Potter, B. Swinburn, J. Schultz, and M. Lawrence. 2010. Prioritizing policy interventions to improve diets? Will it work, can it happen, will it do harm? *Health Promotion International* 25(1):123-133.

Steinbrook, R. 2008. Saying no isn't nice: The travails of Britain's National Institute for Health and Clinical Excellence. *New England Journal of Medicine* 359(19):1977-1981.

Stufflebeam, D. L. 1999. *Foundational models for 21st Century program evaluation.* Kalamazoo, MI: Evaluation Center, Western Michigan University.

Subcommittee on Evaluation Standards. 1958. *Proposed practices for economic analysis of river basin projects.* Washington, DC: Inter-Agency Committee on Water Resources.

UCLA HIA-CLIC (University of California, Los Angeles, Health Impact Assessment-Clearinghouse Learning and Information Center). 2012. *Phases of HIA: 2. Scoping.* http://www.hiaguide.org/methods-resources/methods/phases-hia-2-scoping (accessed May 22, 2012).

U.S. Preventive Services Task Force. 2012. *Procedure manual (USPSTF).* http://www.uspreventiveservicestaskforce.org/uspstf08/methods/procmanual3.htm (accessed May 21, 2012).

Watson, M. R., A. M. Horowitz, I. Garcia, and M. T. Canto. 2001. A community participatory oral health promotion program in an inner-city Latino community. *Journal of Public Health Dentistry* 61(1):34-41.

Weinstein, M. C., and W. B. Stason. 1977. Foundations of cost-effectiveness analysis for health and medical practices. *New England Journal of Medicine* 296(13):716-721.

Weisbrod, B. A. 1983. A guide to benefit-cost analysis, as seen through a controlled experiment in treating the mentally ill. *Journal of Health Politics, Policy and Law* 7(4):808-845.

Woolf, S. H., C. G. Husten, L. S. Lewin, J. Marks, J. Fielding, and E. Sanchez. 2009. *The economic argument for disease prevention: Distinguishing between value and savings.* Washington, DC: Partnership for Prevention.

5

A Framework for Assessing the Value of Community-Based Prevention

This chapter proposes and describes a framework for assessing the value of community-based prevention. It addresses the need to take a comprehensive view of benefits and resources used, which is central to recognizing the far-reaching effects of community-based prevention; it proposes the development of summary measures to support a comprehensive perspective; it explains the need to base valuation on changes in benefits and resources used; and it describes the prospective use of the framework for decision making, and its retrospective use to evaluate programs and policies once they have been implemented. The chapter then reviews the data needed to quantify value within this framework along with the limitations of the data, discusses how communities and other stakeholders can use the framework to value community-based prevention, and concludes with a discussion of the implications for state and national policy.

A FRAMEWORK FOR ASSESSING VALUE

Existing frameworks for community-based prevention interventions neglect one or more of the elements previously identified as being key to the success of such a framework. In this chapter the committee assembles various elements of existing frameworks into a new framework that measures in a way that suits the unique aspects of community-based prevention.

The goals of this framework are (1) to incorporate the full scope of benefits into the value of interventions so that in addition to health benefits and harms, the benefits and harms from community well-being and community process are included; (2) to emphasize that value requires a comparison of the benefits and harms of an intervention with the resources used for that intervention; (3) allow the specific characteristics and context of individual communities to be reflected in the valuation of community-based prevention; (4) to promote the quantification of value in terms of projected or actual changes due to the intervention; and (5) to encourage the development of evidence so as to make understanding the effects of interventions easier and more reliable.

The committee's proposed framework for assessing the value of community-based prevention is shown in schematic form in Figure 5-1. For the assessment of value, the framework proposes a comprehensive consideration of benefits and harms in the context of health, community well-being, and community process as well as an inclusive and comprehensive consideration of the resources used.

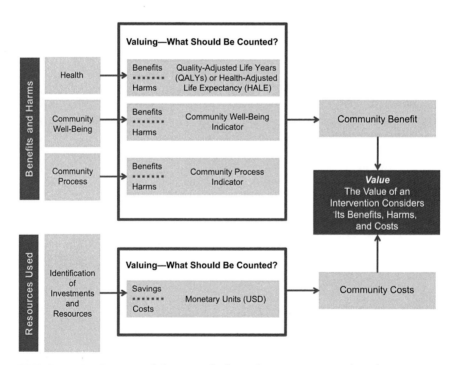

FIGURE 5-1 Conceptual framework for valuing community-based prevention interventions.

The Framework Should Take a Comprehensive View

To value an intervention one should take into account its outcomes (i.e., benefits and harms), the resources used in the intervention itself, and the downstream costs and savings. The valuation of community-based prevention interventions should take a comprehensive perspective—that is, that the measurement of benefits, harms, and resources should include impacts on all members of the community as well as on stakeholders who may be outside the community.

There are many stakeholders involved in community-based prevention, each of which is likely to be impacted differently: individuals, families, communities, businesses, taxpayers, and governments at the local, state, and federal level. It can be helpful to assess value from one or more of these other perspectives, but those assessments should be presented and considered relative to the comprehensive perspective. For example, if an intervention is federally funded but the benefits occur locally, the value of the intervention from the perspective of the community will be greater than its value from the federal perspective because the community does not pay all the costs of the intervention. Good decisions will be based on information about benefits and costs to all stakeholders.

To support a comprehensive framework and focus attention on the breadth of benefits that such a framework encompasses, the committee proposes that benefits be grouped into the three broad categories of health, community well-being, and community process, as discussed in Chapter 3. The measurement of benefits and harms should occur in all three areas. Resources used are a fourth major category of consequences to be considered in valuing community-based prevention. This comprehensive perspective should be the reference point in decision making.

> **Recommendation 1: The committee recommends that those seeking to assign value to community-based prevention interventions take a comprehensive view that includes the benefits and harms in the three major domains of health, community well-being, and community process as well as the resource use associated with such interventions.**

Table 5-1 provides a summary of the proposed framework compared to the eight existing frameworks discussed in Chapter 4.

Proposed Summary Measures

There are a variety of sources of data on health, including surveys (e.g., the National Health Interview Survey and the Behavioral Risk Factor Surveillance System), cohort studies (e.g., the Framingham Heart Study),

TABLE 5-1   Nine Frameworks Summarized

	Includes Comprehensive Set of Valued Outcomes	Compares Benefits with Costs	Accounts for Differences Among Communities
Benefit–cost analysis	Yes, can account for all benefits	Yes	Low; can account for context
Cost-effectiveness analysis	No, health only	Yes	Low; can account for context
Congressional Budget Office scoring	No, only federal spending and revenue	Yes	Low; designed for Congressional budget process
PRECEDE–PROCEED framework	No, although it includes both health and community process	No	High; used in communities
RE-AIM framework	No, health only	No	High; used by evaluators
Health Impact Assessment framework	No, health only	No	High; used in communities
Community Preventive Services Task Force guidelines	No, health only	No	Moderate; focus on community
Lomas model	No, valued outcomes not specified	No	Moderate; focus on decision-making process
Proposed framework	Yes	Yes	High; involves communities in process

registries, health services data, and vital statistics and data collected by state public health agencies. Unfortunately, there are several limitations when attempting to use these data for local, community-based measurement (IOM, 2011). Identifying measures and sources of information for community well-being and community process elements is even more challenging than identifying these items for health. Such efforts will require an increased focus on identifying appropriate information gaps and data sources.

> **Recommendation 2: The committee recommends that the CDC**
> a. develop an inventory of existing data sources for health, community well-being, and community process;
> b. identify gaps in data sources; and
> c. develop data sources to fill those gaps.

Different metrics are appropriate for measuring the different domains of value. Chapter 3 describes many of the outcomes that can be important in each domain. Health impacts, for example, can be measured by changes in intermediate outcomes such as blood pressure or weight, by changes in the numbers of cases of disease, or by changes in health-related quality of life, the numbers of deaths, or quality-adjusted life years (QALYs). Community well-being encompasses an even wider range of possible outcomes and measures. Community process adds another set. The resources used for community-based interventions—and any savings that may result from them—add still another set. Choosing among community-based prevention policies and pro-grams can be difficult when programs have so many effects and those effects take so many different forms. The larger the menu of interventions, and the larger the number of valued outcomes, the more difficult choices become. Decision makers can end up focusing on one outcome, such as health, and ignoring others simply because it is too difficult to take them all into account. A few overall metrics can help prevent this narrowing of focus.

The committee proposes that four metrics be developed to assess the value of community-based prevention: changes in health, changes in com-munity well-being, changes in community process, and changes in resources used.

Health outcomes in the population can be valued with QALYs or health-adjusted life expectancy (HALE). These metrics are well developed and widely used. Each incorporates important domains such as physical well-being, mental well-being, role function, and social function.

The committee is unaware of generally accepted single metrics for the domains of community well-being and community process, although a set of relevant elements and an algorithm for each could be developed similar to those used for the "EuroQol," Quality of Well Being, or the Health Utility Index for health-related quality of life. Measures of community well-being, such as the Urban Hardship Index[1] and the Community Well-Being (CWB) indices (e.g., the Canadian Arctic CWB Index[2]), or the county health rankings could serve as starting points, but they have significant limitations in scope.

The committee recognizes that developing these single indicators is a complex task that will require expertise from outside of the field of health. The committee also recognizes that the development of the single indicator is a long-term goal, since such indicators do not currently exist for the com-munity well-being and community process domains. The National Preven-tion, Health Promotion, and Public Health Council (Prevention Council) is

---

[1] See http://www.rockinst.org/pdf/cities_and_neighborhoods/2004-08-an_update_on_urban_hardship.pdf.

[2] See http://www.aadnc-aandc.gc.ca/eng/1100100016579.

an interagency group established by the Affordable Care Act and chaired by the Surgeon General. The Prevention Council recognizes that the health of a community is influenced by a number of factors outside of the health care and public health sectors, including education, housing, and transportation. Such a group is well positioned to encourage the research needed in the multiple sectors that need to be involved in developing a community benefit indicator.

> **Recommendation 3: The committee recommends that the National Prevention, Health Promotion, and Public Health Council and other public and private sponsors support research aimed at developing**
> a. **a single metric for appraising a community's well-being,**
> b. **a single metric for appraising community processes, and**
> c. **a single metric for combining indicators of community well-being and community process with health into a single indicator of community benefit that can be considered in the context of costs and used to determine the value of a community-based prevention intervention.**

The committee envisions a well-being and process index that is roughly parallel to QALYs and HALE for health. QALYs and HALE can account for differences in how people value health and other outcomes, much as can be done with willingness to pay (WTP). QALYs calculate not just years of life saved but the quality of each life year as determined by an elicitation of preferences. QALY weights can be determined using community, individual, or patient preferences depending upon the context of the analysis. In addition, QALYs are specific to the desired outcome of the intervention. For example, QALYs used to compare an intervention aimed at lowering blood pressure would be different from an intervention aimed at reducing automobile injuries. The QALY is a common single indicator that can be used in many different contexts (Gold et al., 1996).

Likewise, HALE is also a measure of both duration and quality of life. According to a previous IOM committee (2011) HALE weights "have the ability to take into account the effects of particular illnesses; provide insight into regional differences associated with social, environmental, and behavioral risk factors; and allow examination of the health experiences of subpopulations by race/ethnicity." In other words, HALE can account for differences in preferences and population.

Although recognizing the challenges, it is worth pursuing the development of a single indicator that can aid in valuing community well-being as well as an indicator for community process. These indicators, like QALYs and HALE, would combine objective measures of well-being and process status with subjective measures of preference.

Multi-Attribute Utility (MAU) and the Analytic Hierarchy Process (AHP) are examples of methodologies that can be used to develop the community well-being, community process, and community benefit metrics. Health-Related Quality of Life (HRQoL) is a set of metrics that is used to value the multiple dimensions of health, such as mental function, physical function, and role function, and to combine them into a single, preference-based measure, such as the Quality of Well-Being (QWB), Health Utilities Index (HUI), and EuroQoL. They were developed using MAU techniques, much the same as used for other complex decision models such as those for assessing business decisions and defense strategies. The same approach can be used to identify key components of community well-being and to value them. The MAU approach "combines multiple attributes, such as health, equity and empowerment, by eliciting importance (trade-off) weights for attributes" (Peacock et al., 2007). The six steps in the methodology are to (1) identify relevant attributes; (2) describe the levels of the attributes (for example, civic participation could be described as active involvement, medium involvement, low involvement); (3) the levels within each attribute are scaled from 1-100; (4) the attributes are assessed in terms of their relative importance; (5) an intervention is evaluated in terms of how well it contributes to each relevant attribute; and (6) scores are combined to calculate the combined benefit score (Peacock et al., 2007). The AHP is a method used to arrange options in a hierarchy in order to assist in decision making. The steps in the AHP are similar to those of MAU, and include breaking down the decision into interrelated decision elements (for example, the elements within each domain affected by an intervention); "collecting data by pair-wise comparisons of the decision elements"; and estimating the relative weights of the decision elements (Zahedi, 1986). As applied to community well-being, the steps would include identifying the components that the community values, such as aesthetics, ability to meet basic needs, and resilience; developing a scale for each; and then to value (weight) each of the components. One can then assess interventions based on their ability to affect each of the components and combine them into a total "score" so that interventions can be compared.

Unlike the health domain, which has developed the QALY and the HALE, a single metric does not currently exist for the domain of community well-being nor does a single metric exist for the domain of community process. Therefore, other options must be used until such time as those metrics are developed. It is reasonable to consider using a mixture of quantitative and qualitative approaches. Such a mixed model would allow for an action-oriented approach to reach a quantifiable solution. That is, the mixed model may provide information that ultimately will inform how to come to such a solution.

Measures of the built and natural environments; and measures of education, crime, employment, and equity; and various other elements of interest could be combined into a measure of overall community well-being by weighting the changes produced by an intervention in the component outcomes by the community's preferences for each specific outcome. Similarly an aggregate measure for the process-related benefits could be developed that would reflect the value placed on the way that deliberations occur regarding community-based programs and policies, about the manner in which decisions are made and reported, and the manner in which community-based interventions are implemented. Box 5-1 provides an example.

BOX 5-1
Valuing the Construction of a Greenway
Using the Proposed Framework

A community concerned about obesity is looking for ways to encourage more physical activity. One proposal is to convert unused public land along a mass transit corridor into a greenway with a series of pedestrian and bike trails along with other recreational facilities, as several other cities throughout the United States have done or proposed to do. The greenway would pass through several different communities, some affluent and some poor, linking diverse parts of the city.

Using the framework, each affected community as well as other stakeholders would have to decide which outcomes or elements it valued within the proposed three domains of health, community well-being, and community process. Improved health could be one possible outcome and there is ample evidence that increased physical activity leads to better health in the long term. This may be the outcome of highest priority for potential funders, such as government agencies or private foundations. But taking a comprehensive view, as recommended by the committee could lead to the identification of other valued outcomes. For example, for one community the greenway has the potential to improve the communities aesthetically as well as to provide greater opportunity for social and community engagement. This community may value increased recreation facilities more than any other outcome. City leaders may value the development of under-utilized land and the addition of amenities to the city. In addition, the greenway could provide an alternate transportation path that could decrease the number of trips made by cars, thereby improving air quality and decreasing traffic. Finally, the construction of the greenway provides local communities with the opportunity to participate in the implementation of a project that reflects their preferences and values, thereby promoting community empowerment.

Along with the potential benefits, however, there are potential harms. Pedestrians and cyclists on the path face a risk of injury. Members of the various communities would be inconvenienced and annoyed by the construction of the greenway and they may find that their differing preferences and values lead to conflict at the planning level. Moreover, communities may find that the placement of recreational facilities or some other aspect of building the greenway creates or

The resources used for an intervention can be summarized in dollars or other currency. As presented in the framework, costs are inclusive of goods and services purchased in markets—what everyone recognizes as costs because money must be paid out—and also donated goods and services. As a comprehensive summary measure, these costs could be captured and represented as a "Community Costs" indicator and used in arriving at the value of an intervention.

Given that the outcomes in the four domains are—or will be once they are developed—measured in different units, it is currently not possible to provide a single widely-used indicator of the value of community-based

highlights disparities in the distribution of resources between communities. Some communities may fear that the greenway will bring strangers or outsiders into their community and make it less desirable.

All of these potential benefits and harms should be identified and weighed by the communities and decision makers considering the proposal. For the health benefits and harms, measures such as QALYs and HALE offer well-established means of valuation. In the community well-being and community process domains there are no universally accepted measures. Until these measures are developed there is value in community identification of the constituent benefits and harms because this allows the community to consider the full range of consequences of the proposed intervention. For example, as discussed in Chapter 3, there are positive outcomes in perceived general health associated with access to green space. A shift in transportation preferences away from car trips could, over time, lead to better outdoor air quality. From these projected changes from the current baseline, decision makers could derive an idea of the potential net community benefit even if widely accepted summary measures of community well-being and community process are currently unavailable.

In addition to identifying the benefits and harms of the intervention within the three domains, communities and decision makers must also identify the costs of the intervention. As discussed in Chapter 3 the costs of an intervention should be considered from a comprehensive perspective in order to encourage a full accounting and to discourage double counting. The costs of the proposed greenway would include the short-term capital outlay for construction and landscaping and long-term maintenance and security costs. They would also include the costs of unpaid volunteer time within the community for maintaining and managing the greenway. There are widely accepted methods of capturing these costs and expressing them using a common metric.

After determining the community benefit and the community cost, decision makers are in a better position to value the proposed intervention. In addition, they can determine which indicators will be valuable in evaluating the intervention. Many of the projected benefits of the greenway will not occur for a number of years, such as lowering obesity rates. Thus, the time horizons used in valuing the greenway must be appropriate for the valued outcomes. Decision makers should take this into account when valuing and evaluating the intervention.

prevention. However, once a single indicator of Community Benefit is developed, it should be considered alongside the Community Cost indicator, and value could be expressed as units of Community Benefit per dollar. It should be noted that if the community benefit indicator is determined to be negative, no further valuation need be conducted. Summary measures for each of the three domains of benefit and for resources used are a first step toward a possible future overall summary measure.

Valuation Is Based on Changes in Benefits and Costs

Value is based on *changes* relative to some baseline or to an alternative intervention. The value of a community-based prevention intervention reflects its impacts relative to what would have happened in its absence or relative to an alternative community-based prevention intervention. Changes due to adding an intervention are usually referred to as incremental changes, whereas applying an existing intervention more intensively is usually referred to as a marginal change. In principle, the assessment of the value of an intervention should include changes in everything that has a reasonable chance of changing by more than a trivial amount as a result of the intervention or its intensification.

It is important to assess the actual changes that are projected to occur as a result of an intervention and to express them in absolute terms, such as QALYs or HALE, rather than in relative terms, such as a percentage change. Stakeholders often assess the value of an intervention in terms of the overall burden of the health problem or the size of the effect of an intervention. However, these metrics are, by themselves, inadequate for measuring value since they do not consider the overall health impact of an intervention. A problem may be large, but if none of the available interventions is effective against it, then they have little value despite the size of the problem; similarly, an intervention may have a large effect size (e.g., it may reduce an adverse health impact by 90 percent), but if the number of individuals affected is very small, then the overall health impact will be small as well. The preventable burden (effectiveness times size of the problem) is a better measure of impact than either the effect size or the size of the affected population considered alone.

Recommendation 4: The committee recommends that those assessing value should include in their assessments the expected or demonstrated changes, both positive and negative, that result from the intervention.

Prospective Assessment for Decision Making

The central task of the framework is to support decision making about choices and options between various possible community-based prevention interventions. An assessment of the value of an intervention can be prospective (before the intervention occurs) so as to inform decisions about which interventions to choose, or concurrent (while the intervention is ongoing), or retrospective (after the intervention concludes) to inform decisions about whether and how to continue an intervention.

The prospective assessment of the value of an intervention requires three steps: (1) the identification of factors that are valued by the community, (2) projection of the changes in outcomes (impact) expected as a result of the proposed intervention and of the resources to be used, and (3) estimation of the value of the projected changes. Each step is critical to estimating the value of an intervention for the purpose of decision making. Each step is explored below.

Understanding what the community cares about in each of the three domains (health, community well-being, and community process) is critical for designing and proposing interventions that address areas of importance to the community. This assessment will not only identify important health (and non-health) factors in the community, but it will also identify those factors for which improvement is preferred by community members. What is important for one community may not be important for another.

Recommendation 5: The committee recommends that those involved in decision making ensure that the elements included in valuing community-based prevention interventions reflect the preferences of an inclusive range of stakeholders.

The second step is the projection of changes. This includes both the projected costs of the intervention itself and the benefits, including savings, and harms that are projected to occur as a result. To support good decisions it is essential to list all the outcomes of importance and to show how much each intervention contributes to each outcome. Health is usually projected in terms of intermediate outcomes, such as changes in weight or blood pressure, cases of disease, and deaths, and it can be summarized, as noted earlier, by QALYs gained, or by HALE. Community well-being might be measured by reductions in crime using statistics already established by police systems, by increases in educational attainment, by additions to green space, or through surveys of how people feel about their community and the changes in it. Community process might be measured, very roughly, by the number of people participating in local planning activities or the hours of work volunteered in a year, or, more carefully through surveys that ask people in what ways and how much, beyond the consequences for health, they value the activities in which they participate or the transparency with which the decisions are made. Indicators for these two domains do not yet exist and the committee recommends their development (Recommendation 3).

Program costs—the resources used in implementing the policy or strategy—should also be projected. All resources used should be projected, regardless of the source of funds used to purchase them or whether they are non-monetary, such as donated time. In this framework the committee specifically recognizes that context (which includes the implementation process, the determinants of health, and the community's characteristics) is critical to the success and thus to the projected impact of the intervention. The focus on intervention context encourages those engaged in the valuing process to recognize that community-based prevention can be a complex system within which prevention policies, programs, determinants, stakeholders, and strategies interact dynamically.

The third step is the estimation of the value of the projected changes. Once community members have listed all the outcomes they value and measured the effects of interventions in those terms, they have to choose among interventions. That can be hard to do when the valued outcomes take different forms. Policy A may provide safer streets and community participation among parents and children. Strategy B may provide meals and social interaction for isolated elderly people. Interventions C, D, and E may offer still other things of value. Which are most valuable? Which should be done if not all can be? Which should be done first? Valuation typically involves assigning weights to the projected changes or ranking the changes, in order to summarize the value of an intervention.

If there are only a few choices and only a few valued outcomes, listing the contributions of each intervention to each outcome, as described in step 2, can be sufficient to allow people to choose among them. But the larger the menu of choices, and the larger the number of valued outcomes, the more difficult the choice becomes. In that case people can end up focusing on one outcome, such as health, and ignoring the others simply because it becomes too difficult to take them all into account. As noted, a single indicator can help prevent this narrowing of focus. The three domains of value recommended by the committee are a step in the direction of the necessary summary measures.

Cost–benefit analysis offers one approach to summarizing benefits (and costs). In the cost–benefit approach all the individual components are converted to dollar values. However, because many people are reluctant to convert health outcomes into dollars and because of the challenge in valuing intangible benefits and harms such as social and environmental changes and changes in process, it may be desirable to develop several intermediate indicators, as recommended by the committee. These indicators will make it possible to reduce the important outcomes of community-based prevention to a more manageable—but still understandable—number. In either case the goal is to encourage the adoption of interventions for which the value of the benefits exceeds the value of the resources required to produce them.

Re-Valuation

Prospective valuation feeds directly into the process of deciding whether or not to allocate resources, which may require deciding among priorities competing for the same resources. If the decision is not to invest, the process ends there. If the decision is to invest in the proposed community-based prevention intervention, the process continues with the implementation of the program in the community. While the framework for valuing is complete at this point, implementation should be accompanied by an evaluation of the intervention's performance and of how well it delivers value to the community, as well as by ongoing monitoring and reporting of progress. The ultimate effects of an intervention depend on the quality of its design and implementation. Context is a powerful determinant of the ultimate outcomes and practice-based evidence of effectiveness becomes an important source of data for those contemplating investment of resources in other communities (Pronk, 2012). Evaluation, which can be thought of as re-valuation, is thus key. For example, the effect of a given initiative could change over time. It could become stronger as community norms and expectations change, as in the decreasing acceptability of smoking in public spaces. Or it could become weaker as the initial enthusiasm for a change wears off, as with the fitness initiatives of the early 1960s.

The evaluation process follows projection processes closely. In particular, as the program or policy is in operation and actual resources are being used for it one component of evaluation focuses on quantifying the results of the program. Measurement includes an assessment of the resources actually deployed and the extent to which the projected changes in intermediate and long-term outcomes are achieved. The duration of the intervention may affect its costs. Fixed costs and variable, recurring costs should both be considered, with appropriate discounting. For example, a school-based educational campaign will need to be repeated for each new cohort of students; the fixed costs of developing the curriculum can be spread over the years it is used. When both costs and benefits—and, therefore, their ratio to each other or the costs relative to added years (or added quality) of life—can vary over time, it is important to include time in the evaluation of the intervention.

Measurement of the baseline state before the intervention is also required so that changes may be determined at intermediate steps in the process of implementing the intervention or after completion. For example, it is important to know if necessary resources were mobilized across the community and to what degree the intervention was applied to the target audience(s). Measurements should be made across all the factors in the health, community well-being, and community process domains that were previously identified by the community as being valued. Including such an examination in the evaluation process also provides information that can be used to determine how well the framework accurately projected change.

The evaluation component considers the short-, intermediate-, and long-term impacts of the community-based prevention intervention and provides ongoing reports of progress over time. Program administrators should consider how this intervention may be assessed in terms of its implementation fidelity (the degree of fit between the developer-defined elements of a prevention program and its actual implementation in a given organization or community setting), how it may be generalized to other audiences or communities, whether or not the intervention is scalable and sustainable in the long run, and how to share what is learned of the actual process of implementation with others so that this knowledge can be disseminated as practice-based evidence of effectiveness. Finally, ongoing reporting of experience and progress should be shared with all stakeholders, used for continuous improvement, and aligned with surveillance efforts of health indicators across the community.

INFORMATION NEEDED TO ASSESS
VALUE USING THIS FRAMEWORK

According to the way that the committee has presented the framework, there are three types of information needed to assess the value of an intervention: (1) What is the baseline state? (2) What impacts might an intervention have? (3) What impacts did an intervention have? The answers to all three questions should represent the best information available. In Chapter 4 the committee noted the importance of being explicit about the data sources and criteria for admissible evidence to be used in the assessment of value.

One important methodological note is that formal program evaluation requires a reasonable way to determine what the progress in those outcomes would have been had the intervention not taken place. Measurement of a baseline is needed in order to project such changes or to measure the relative impact of intervention implementations at various times. Baseline measurement needs to occur in the health, community well-being, and community process domains and, ideally, be reflected in the summary measures proposed. Therefore, the committee urges that evaluations include a reasonable control or comparison group or other methodology (interrupted time series, quantitative and qualitative mixed methods, etc.) to support the evaluation of the impact of the intervention.

Systematic literature reviews on the evidence of effectiveness provide the highest quality information for projecting changes in outcomes, but other sources are often needed, particularly when estimating the value of interventions prospectively. Good-quality cost data are also important (Luce et al., 1996; Polsky and Glick, 2009). As empirical evidence accumulates, that information can be used to refine the analyses.

Information related to the impact of the intervention should be considered in the context of a model of causation (or a logic framework) that allows the outcomes valued by the community to be connected (both positively and negatively) to the various activities included in the intervention. For example, the causal loop subsystem related to tobacco use prevention policies described in Appendix B specifies a variety of factors important in generating changes. Based on this type of approach, information may be gathered that is, at a minimum, inclusive of the factors outlined in the causal model.

HOW TO USE THE FRAMEWORK IN
THE COMMUNITY CONTEXT

An assessment of the value of an intervention is just one piece within the larger decision-making process. The proposed framework is intended to aid decision making about adopting community-based prevention interventions in a broad range of contexts. It is also intended to assist in the task of monitoring and evaluating community-based prevention interventions once they have been adopted and implemented. Decision makers may operate at the level of higher-level funders, whether public (national or state agencies) or private (foundations or businesses), or they may operate at the level of a community initially deciding what to propose to a local government or to a decision maker at a higher level considering competing proposals. At any level, an early decision must be made about the group of stakeholders that should be included in the process of planning and valuing the proposal. Although who should be included will vary with the nature of the intervention and the level at which the decision about adoption will be made, in general a broader group of decision makers will give voice to a broader range of values to be considered. The framework encourages a comprehensive valuation process and so encourages the broad inclusion of various stakeholders in a decision. Furthermore, the different voices need to be balanced so that some stakeholders do not have undue influence at the expense of others.

The framework encourages a broad consideration of the benefits and harms as well as the costs of a community-based prevention intervention. It seeks some agreement on the net benefit or value of any intervention while recognizing two prominent features of the situation that make such agreement on its value something that may take thoughtful deliberation by decision makers, including some negotiation and compromise. The two features are that there is often disagreement about just what values must be considered; the second is that some of the values may be difficult to quantify, making it difficult to compare them and arrive at agreement. These are unavoidable features of a situation with a range of kinds of benefits, kinds of costs, and kinds of harms.

Accordingly, the framework does not offer a decision procedure or algorithm for making choices about competing interventions. The framework nevertheless can help decision makers and others identify the types of outcomes that contribute to the value of an intervention. If the intervention is setting aside lane space for bicycling, for example, there are quantifiable health effects, not only from the exercise, but also from the reduction of bicycling accidents. There may also be non-quantifiable effects of people bicycling, such as the pleasure of activity and the respect for those engaged in it that is shown by setting aside space for it. The framework reminds deliberators to think about the broad range of valued consequences of the community-based prevention intervention.

One dimension of the health outcomes that affects value is the possible conflict between equity and improving aggregate health for a population. Sometimes these two goals of health policy pull in the same direction, and sometimes they conflict. A community-based prevention intervention may be good at improving aggregate health, but it may have a greater effect on those already better off in some important way—say by income or residential location or occupational status—and this may increase health disparities. The willingness of people to trade off increased inequality for aggregate improvement may vary significantly. Reasonable disagreement about how to weigh these two values may persist, and the framework can make the source of that disagreement more visible.

Furthermore, community-based interventions often focus their gains and harms on particular groups within a community. Likely targets of an intervention include people with low income, people with disabilities, and racial and ethnic minorities. An important question is whether or not special weight should be given to gains or harms accruing to or imposed on particular groups. If particular communities prefer to attach special import to the gains or harms that accrue to certain target groups, efforts should be made to establish explicit weights that could be attached to these gains and harms. In this way, the desire to reflect equity concerns in the valuation effort can be achieved in the overall valuation process. However, it is important that the process be clear and explicit. This requires that a clear set of weights or values be established before attaching the weights to the projections of gains and harms to particular groups.

The persistence of such disagreement around values suggests there may be a legitimacy problem for decision makers. Even if they are the appropriate authorities for making such decisions, they need to make them in the "right" way if legitimacy is to be obtained. They must listen to the appropriate voices expressing different value commitments. Their process should search for rationales that take the relevant values into consideration, and the rationales must explain the basis for giving them the weight that the decision reflects. The framework can help identify the value components that need to be considered, and it can even help clarify who might value those issues and therefore who should be listened to. Applying the framework to alternative interventions may thus clarify the various ways in which the value of these interventions differs. As stated above, the committee recommends that the value of community-based prevention interventions should reflect the preferences of an inclusive range of stakeholders.

Transparency improves the deliberative process, and the framework emphasizes its importance. Determining the value of an intervention in a transparent way can enhance legitimacy. In particular, it is important that the rationales for decisions be made publicly available.

The framework can also be used in revisiting a decision in light of new evidence and arguments. In this context it can add consistency to the deliberation by helping decision makers consider again the range of values that influenced the original decision.

Monitoring and evaluation of an intervention can answer the question, does the value it initially promised and that was the basis for adopting it emerge in the process of implementation? The framework can guide the design of monitoring and evaluation that should be part of good planning for any community-based prevention intervention. The comprehensive identification of the specific benefits, harms, and resources used that were included in the value of the intervention should guide the monitoring and evaluation process, for it will track the resulting intervention to see if estimated net benefits are realized. Ideally, a good monitoring and evaluation process can identify ways to improve the implementation or revise the intervention so that negative effects, or costs can be reduced. The framework urges such ongoing assessment of the value of a community-based prevention intervention.

Recommendation 6: The committee recommends that, to assure transparency,

a. analysts make publicly available the evidence used for valuation and provide estimates of the uncertainty of their results, and
b. decision makers make publicly available the rationale for their decisions.

IMPLICATIONS FOR STATE AND NATIONAL POLICY

Frameworks for valuation, such as the one presented in this paper, have the potential to impact federal, state, and local policy making in significant ways. Chapter 4 reviewed eight existing valuation frameworks: benefit–cost analysis, cost-effectiveness analysis, Congressional Budget Office scoring, the PRECEDE–PROCEED framework, the RE-AIM framework, Health Impact Assessment, the Community Preventive Services Task Force guidelines, and the Canadian Health Services Research Foundation (Lomas) model. These eight frameworks have several elements in common: (1) They have passed through many rounds of validation and refinement, (2) they are broadly accepted among researchers and policy makers, and (3) they are incorporated into the formal process of policy making and not merely used piecemeal to advocate for or against specific proposals.

As with the frameworks discussed in Chapter 4, the committee's framework has limitations. The framework presented in this report is in its very early stages, and so its near-term impact on policy making is likely limited. Because of the importance of contextual factors and the limited scope and generalizability of evidence on the effects of community-based prevention, the framework does not yet provide a detailed roadmap for valuation. Clear, consistent measurement of the elements of value are important. Yet comprehensive data are often not available to measure tangible benefits adequately and the measurement of the many intangible benefits is not yet well developed. Such a broadly inclusive framework may seem overly abstract or unreliable to some observers. As the framework is applied, new measures and data sources will need to be developed as will an appropriate methodology for creating valid single indicators for community well-being and community process. Old measures and data sources will need to be applied in new ways, a process that will take time to establish validity and gain acceptance. The committee has recommended several steps to take to promote progress on these fronts. Although much work remains, the committee's proposed framework is designed to capture the value of community-based prevention by taking a comprehensive approach, comparing benefits, harms, and resources used in three domains, and taking into account community context.

Expanding the influence of this framework will require building a consensus that the outcomes on which it focuses (health, community well-being, community process, and resources used) are broadly important and not just the narrow interests of a specific group. First and foremost, such validation involves testing whether or not this model is useful to communities and stakeholders in general as an organizing framework. Next, one would need to examine how the framework, in general, responds to such factors as utility, feasibility, propriety, and accuracy. Furthermore, validation of the framework could include a consideration of its scalability and sustainability, whether it can support capacity building for health in communities, whether it can address health equity effectively, and whether it is generalizable across many contexts and settings.

It will also be important to validate the framework by showing repeatedly that it correctly distinguishes between interventions that improve community well-being and those that do not. This process of validation will almost certainly require refining the framework and expanding the underlying evidence base. Following consensus and validation, the framework can be formally incorporated into the policy-making process. This formal role could consist of a requirement that legislative or grant proposals be accompanied by an objective impact assessment based on the framework or of a requirement that executive branch agencies use the framework in evaluating the output of their programs. A formal role could also consist of a requirement that discretionary funding be distributed based on valuations that use the framework. Although that type of role may be many years off, the existing frameworks described in Chapter 4 provide clear precedents for such a progression.

CONCLUSION

Two transitions have led to changes in perspective about the kinds of interventions needed to address today's challenges to living a healthy life: (1) the shift in major causes of illness and death from communicable diseases to chronic diseases, and (2) an increased emphasis on the social determinants of health. Community-based prevention interventions seek to address the distribution of health and risk factors in populations (e.g., the social determinants of health) that contribute to today's primary causes of death and disease. But determining the value of community-based interventions has proven difficult. Existing frameworks for valuing interventions fall short, and the committee concluded that what is needed is a framework that focuses on population-level impact and that can take account of intersectoral action, community participation and empowerment, context, and systems thinking.

The framework proposed by the committee is comprehensive and includes the assessment of the benefits, harms, and resource use of community-based prevention interventions in the three major domains of health, community well-being, and community process. The framework also proposes that summary measures or single indicators be developed to assess value in these three areas and that these be compared with a summary measure of resource use. Until such time as a single indicator for each domain exists, however, it will be appropriate to use different metrics for measuring the different domains of value. Chapter 3 describes many of the outcomes that can be measured and weighted in each domain.

The assessment of value of an intervention usually takes place within a decision-making context. Stakeholders and decision makers come from different perspectives and emphasize different factors. It is important, therefore, that the value assessment reflect the preferences of an inclusive range of stakeholders. It is also important that there be transparency in the use of the framework so that there is understanding about the rationale and evidence used for making decisions.

As stated earlier, the proposed framework is in its very early stages and much is yet to be learned. However, the framework identifies critical areas for valuing and the report proposes additional areas where work needs to be undertaken.

REFERENCES

Gold, M., J. Siegel, L. Russell, and M. Weinstein. 1996. *Cost-effectiveness in health and medicine*. New York: Oxford University Press.

IOM (Institute of Medicine). 2011. A nationwide framework for surveillance of cardiovascular and chronic lung diseases. Washington, DC: The National Academies Press.

Luce, B., W. Manning, J. Siegel, and J. Lipscomb. 1996. Estimating costs in cost-effectiveness analysis. In *Cost effectiveness in health and medicine*, edited by M. Gold and J. Siegel. New York: Oxford University Press.

Peacock, S., J. Richardson, R. Carter, and D. Edwards. 2007. Priority setting in health care using Multi-Attribute Utility Theory and Programme Budgeting and Marginal Analysis (PBMA). *Social Science & Medicine* 64(4):897-910.

Polsky, D., and H. Glick. 2009. Costing and cost analysis in randomised trials: Caveat emptor. *Pharmacoeconomics* 27(3):179.

Pronk, N. P. 2012. The power of context: Moving from information and knowledge to practical wisdom for improving physical activity and dietary behaviors. *American Journal of Preventive Medicine* 42(1):103-104.

Zahedi, F. 1986. The analytic hierarchy process—a survey of the method and its applications. *Interfaces* 16(4):96-108.

A

Glossary

Benefits, for purposes of this report, are defined as the outcomes of a community-based preventive intervention that promote or enhance health, community well-being, or community process.

Community, as defined for the purposes of this report, means any group of people who share geographic space, interests, goals, or history. It also includes the built environment, social networks, and the organizations and institutions that sustain the individual and collective life of the community. The committee believes that a community can exist at both a neighborhood and a national level.

Community-based activity is an activity that involves members of the affected community in the planning, development, implementation, and evaluation of programs and strategies.

Community-based prevention, as defined for purposes of this report, takes a population-based approach to programs and policies oriented to preventing the onset of disease, stopping or slowing the progress of disease, reducing or eliminating the negative consequences of disease, increasing healthful behaviors that result in improvements in health and well-being, or decreasing disparities that result in an inequitable distribution of health. Community-based prevention is not primarily based on clinical services although it may involve services provided by health professionals in clinical settings. For purposes of this report, community-based prevention includes both community-based activities and community-placed activities.

Community-based program, as defined for this report, is a coordinated activity or set of activities, such as an educational campaign against smoking, improvements to the built environment to encourage physical activity, or a chronic disease education and awareness campaign to improve self-management, or a combination of such interventions that is undertaken to accomplish a health objective or outcome.

Community participation refers to the engagement of those affected in the process of transforming conditions.

Community-placed activities are activities that are developed without the participation of the affected community at important stages of the project but for which effort is expended to generate community support.

Community process refers to several elements influencing community participation in the decision making as well as the design and implementation associated with community-based interventions. These elements include civic engagement, local leadership development, community representation, trust, skill building, and community history, among others.

Community well-being includes social norms, how people relate to each other and to their surroundings, and how much investment they are willing to make in themselves and in the people around them. Elements of community well-being include wealth, education, employment, safety, transportation, housing, worksites, food, health care, and recreational spaces.

Costs, for purposes of this report, are the resources necessary to implement a community-based preventive intervention and produce its benefits.

Ecological model "assumes that health and well-being are affected by the interaction among multiple determinants including biology, behavior, and the environment" (IOM, 2003, p. 32).

Empowerment refers to the individual or collective capacity to exercise control over the conditions and circumstances that influence health and well-being.

Harms are the non-economic costs of an intervention to a community, for example, the inconvenience and noise of construction of a bike or walking path or an increase in disparities caused by an intervention that helps one segment of the population more than another.

Health promotion "is the process of enabling people to increase control over, and to improve, their health. It moves beyond a focus on individual behaviour towards a wide range of social and environmental interventions" (http://www.who.int/topics/health_promotion/en/). Health promotion approaches engage people and organizations in the transformation process, and their engagement in the process constitutes in itself a desired change.

Intersectoral action refers to an action in which actors from a variety of relevant sectors are engaged and coordinated in the planning, implementation, and governance of interventions.

Intervention, as defined for this report, is an umbrella term used to mean either a program or a policy that has the goal of improving health.

Opportunity cost is a benefit, profit, or value of something that must be given up to acquire or achieve something else. "Since every resource (land, money, time, etc.) can be put to alternative uses, every action, choice, or decision has an associated opportunity cost" (http://www.businessdictionary.com/definition/opportunity-cost.html).

Policy is a rule or set of guidelines, such as nutritional standards for school lunches.

Population health, as defined by Kindig and Stoddart (2003, p. 380), is "the health outcomes of a group of individuals, including the distribution of such outcomes within the group." "These populations often are geographic regions like nations or communities but also can be other groups, like employees, specific ethnic groups, disabled persons, or prisoners."

Present value is "the current worth of a future sum of money or stream of cash flows given a specified rate of return" (http://www.investopedia.com/terms/p/presentvalue.asp#axzz22UfpMoYB).

Social determinants of health are the "conditions in the environments in which people are born, live, learn, work, play, worship, and age that affect a wide range of health, functioning, and quality-of-life outcomes and risks" (http://healthypeople.gov/2020/topicsobjectives2020/overview.aspx?topicid=39).

Social marketing is the application of marketing principles used to sell products to change attitudes and behaviors. "Social marketing seeks to influence social behaviors not to benefit the marketer, but to benefit the target audience and the general society" (http://www.social-marketing.com/Whatis.html).

Strategy is the method through which programs are implemented, such as television advertisements warning of the dangers of smoking, construction of a bike path, or conducting disease management workshops in churches.

Systems science is the study of "dynamic interrelationships of variables at multiple levels of analysis (e.g., from cells to society) simultaneously (often through causal feedback processes), while also studying the impact on the behavior of the system as a whole over time" (http://obssr.od.nih. gov/scientific_areas/methodology/systems_science/index.aspx).

Value of an intervention is defined as its benefits minus its harms and costs.

REFERENCES

IOM (Institute of Medicine). 2003. *Who will keep the public healthy?* Washington, DC: The National Academies Press.

Kindig, D. A., and G. Stoddart. 2003. What is population health? *American Journal of Public Health* 93:366-369.

B

Examples of Systems Science Approaches to Valuing Community-Based Prevention

Under ideal circumstances, there are sufficient data available for all of the domains and elements of value for the development of decision support tools. A systems science model based on these data and on the causal relationships among the variables could simulate or reproduce the impacts of different interventions on the variables in the system as well as the resulting changes to the structure of the system overall.

Yet, as noted in Chapter 2, many of the policy, system, and environmental interventions to reduce chronic and infectious diseases and to promote population health have a limited evidence base with which to work. There are other obstacles as well, including the short-term tenure of policy and decision makers and disagreements about valued outcomes and priorities among local decision makers. For instance, elected officials may have a preference for innovative strategies rather than evidence-based ones because they wish to draw attention to their campaign or platform or highlight their accomplishments while they are still in office. However, such innovations may be difficult to identify and measure in a timely fashion. As another example, representative input from community members may shed light on previous policy successes and failures or other historical trends; however, the voices of many community members are often underrepresented or infrequently assessed and reported.

One way to advance the field is to use qualitative methods to support the generation of systems science maps or diagrams that capture the underlying theories of change and causal structures in the system. See Figure B-1 for a theoretical illustration of a causal loop diagram—i.e., a map—of a

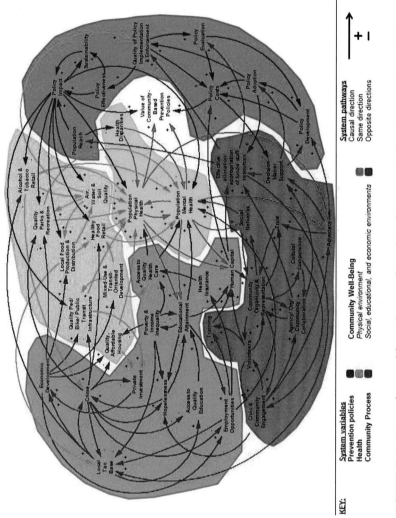
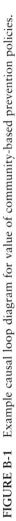

FIGURE B-1 Example causal loop diagram for value of community-based prevention policies.

system that incorporates prevention policies, health, community well-being, and community processes.

Figure B-1 provides an illustration of a comprehensive system for increasing the understanding of the value of community-based prevention policies. While it is difficult to disentangle the multiple moving parts in this comprehensive system, the diagram provides insights about how variables in the system influence or are influenced by multiple other variables in the system (e.g., economic development or population physical health). These variables are cross-cutting variables that appear in multiple pathways emerging from the causal loop diagram, and they highlight important leverage points in the system that can be used to gain momentum for change throughout the system.

Developing these diagrams helps identify variables in the system, causal relationships between the variables in the system, and key leverage points in the system that may impact multiple other variables in the system (e.g., "crime" in Figure B-1). In turn these diagrams can be used to generate common understanding or agreement about the system, to set priorities related to places to intervene in the system, or to identify variables and associated measures that can be assessed in order to test the variables in the system using simulation models, among others. Furthermore, systems science model development efforts benefit from the experiential knowledge that community representatives accumulate about the successes and challenges associated with developing, implementing, and evaluating community-based prevention policies and wellness strategies (Homer and Hirsch, 2006).

A closer examination of the causal loop diagram can also help make more explicit the theories of change—or pathways from prevention policies to health outcomes—as well as the underlying structures serving to reinforce or hinder change processes. See Figure B-2 for an illustration of pathways associated with tobacco use, nutrition, and physical activity.

To understand the feedback loops, it is helpful to take a closer look at some of the pathways in the causal loop diagram in Figure B-2. For example, a feedback loop associated with tobacco use, which is highlighted in yellow, may represent the following causal structure:

- [Start at *Alcohol & Tobacco Retail*] A community with a large number of tobacco outlets has a greater proportion of the population with access to tobacco products, and, consequentially, greater sales of tobacco products;
- [Move to *Population Physical Health*] as members of the community purchase and consume more tobacco products, the rates of heart disease, lung cancer, oral cancer, and other co-morbid conditions associated with tobacco use increase;

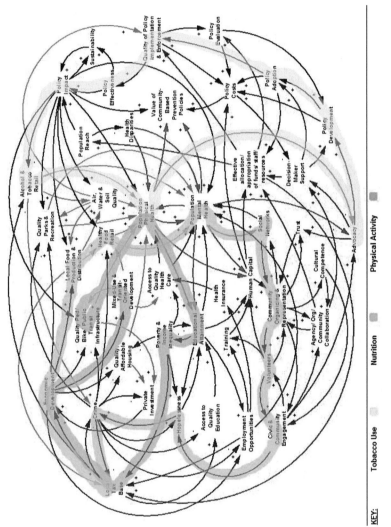

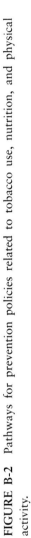

KEY: Tobacco Use   Nutrition   Physical Activity

FIGURE B-2 Pathways for prevention policies related to tobacco use, nutrition, and physical activity.

- [Move to *Advocacy*] with high rates of morbidity and mortality associated with tobacco use, community and health representatives develop advocacy initiatives to draw attention to these serious health concerns;
- [Move to *Policy Development*] advocates support new policies that place restrictions on the sale and distribution of tobacco products or tobacco use, or both;
- [Move to *Policy Adoption*] these policies require buy-in and support from elected officials, who may be influenced by tobacco lobbyists or financial support from the tobacco industry, resulting in potential elimination or dilution of policies;
- [Move to *Quality Policy Implementation & Enforcement*] once a policy is passed, local decision makers also decide on the funding and resources to be allocated to implementation and enforcement of the policy, and, with fewer resources, quality assurance and compliance often suffers;
- [Move to *Policy Effectiveness*] yet, with a rigorous policy in place and resources to support its enforcement, the policy can be efficacious in minimizing the concentration of tobacco outlets, reducing tobacco sales, and decreasing tobacco use;
- [Move to *Policy Impact*] thus, with an increase in these evidence-based policies, the policies are typically replicated in other communities; and
- [Go back to *Alcohol & Tobacco Retail*] the total number of tobacco outlets is reduced along with subsequent declines in tobacco sales and consumption.

In addition, there are a few relevant pathways (not highlighted) for increasing the value of this community-based prevention policy, including greater policy impact, greater population physical health (or mental health as relevant), and fewer policy costs associated with policy development, adoption, implementation, enforcement, and evaluation.

As another example, one of the feedback loops for nutrition is highlighted in blue, and it may represent the following causal structure:

- [Start at *Local Food Production & Distribution*] An increasing number of school and community gardens as well as urban farms are being developed in a community;
- [Move to *Healthy Food Retail*] community members are selling produce from these gardens and urban farms through farmer's markets and mobile vendors to increase access to locally grown fruits and vegetables in the community;

- [Move to *Population Mental Health*] from the markets and vendors, the entire community has access to healthier foods, reducing stresses associated with food insecurity and increasing mental health benefits associated with consumption of nutritious foods;
- [Move to *Social Networks*] as community members feel better and learn more about the gardens and farms, community participation in the gardens and farms increases, and these places increase opportunities for social interactions with other community members;
- [Move to *Community Organizing & Representation*] because of these social interactions, community members become aware of, and more likely to participate in, events, decisions, and changes happening in the community;
- [Move to *Volunteers*] through community outreach, more in-kind services and resources are generated from the community;
- [Move to *Civic & Community Engagement*] as these social movements form and mobilize, community members become more involved in democratic practices (e.g., voting, attending city council meetings, running for office);
- [Move to *Hopelessness*] with participation in community improvements, community members feel a greater sense of pride in their community and optimism about the future of their community;
- [Move to *Crime*] with this sense of hope and time invested in community improvements, a critical mass of community members becomes less tolerant of crime and other activities that cause people to feel unsafe in their own community;
- [Move to *Local Tax Base*] as a result of less crime and more community improvements, the community begins to attract more businesses and residents, increasing the local tax base;
- [Move to *Economic Development*] with more tax dollars, the community can invest more resources into gardens, farms, farmer's markets, and mobile vendors; and
- [Go back to *Local Food Production & Distribution*] thereby, increase the quality and quantity of local food production and distribution.

A final example, which includes one of the feedback loops for physical activity, is highlighted in green. It has the potential to represent the following causal structure:

- [Start at *Quality Ped/Bike/Public Transit Infrastructure*] A sprawling, car-centric community has few options for multi-modal transportation;

- [Move to *Population Physical Health*] children in the community rely on their parents to drive them in cars to school and other destinations in the community, increasing sedentary time sitting in a car and reducing time in active transportation;
- [Move to *Educational Attainment*] as children are more sedentary, expend less energy, and have poorer health, their attention, focus, and performance in school suffers, which may, in turn, affect their overall educational attainment;
- [Move to *Poverty & Income Inequality*] adolescents or young adults with less than a high school education are more likely to have lower-income jobs or to live in poverty;
- [Move to *Local Tax Base*] with more poverty in the community, residents and businesses tend to leave the community and the local tax base declines;
- [Move to *Economic Development*] resources for economic development also go away;
- [Move to *Mixed-Use & Transit-Oriented Development*] leaving no support for new developments that reduce sprawl and car dependence; and
- [Go back to *Quality Ped/Bike/Public Transit Infrastructure*] stagnation or further decline in the quality of multi-modal transportation options.

Through group model building, innovative community participatory methods of data collection and analysis provide opportunities to develop conceptual models with community representatives that can serve as the basis for the construction of the simulation models (Hovmand et al., 2012; Vennix, 1996, 1999). The use of community-based participatory methods has helped to elucidate complex interactions of social, political, economic, environmental, and health conditions as experienced by community members (Krieger et al., 2002; Lantz et al., 2001; Metzler et al., 2003; Schulz et al., 2002); to establish trusting relationships to increase understanding and insight (Lincoln and Guba, 1985); to foster co-learning and capacity building among all partners (Israel et al., 2005); and to create greater balance between knowledge generation and intervention for the mutual benefit of all partners (Wallerstein, 1999).

Likewise, the resource-based view (RBV) of systems provides a method to examine how differences are ascribed to different kinds of systems or different arrangements of tangible and intangible resources. To examine variation across communities, RBV focuses on the level of key resources in communities and how they are arranged (Morecroft, 2008; Morecroft et al., 2002; Warren, 2002). Therefore, differences in trends between systems get explained both by differences in tangible or intangible resources and differences in how those resources are organized. For example, two communities can have the same level of resources (e.g., funding to support air, water, and soil quality), yet exhibit very different trends because the communities differ in how those resources are organized and mobilized (e.g., allocation of funds to policy development, industry regulation, or community promotional campaigns) (Brennan et al., no date).

Tangible resources may include new policies (e.g., a smoking ban or Medicaid reimbursement rules), environments (e.g., farmer's market or mobile health clinics), programs (e.g., the Walking School Bus or after-school programs), promotional efforts (e.g., pink ribbons for breast cancer awareness and condom distribution), and social determinants (e.g., education, housing, and employment), among others. Intangible resources may include engagement (e.g., citizen participation and leadership by local champions), awareness and demand, social norms and influence (e.g., reciprocity and power), and cultural and psychosocial factors (e.g., values and traditions, beliefs). From a practice perspective, tangible resources tend to be easier than intangible resources for decision makers to identify and manage (Morecroft, 2002). In turn, from an evaluation perspective tangible resources are more readily observed and measured, and intangible resources may not get captured in the data or subsequent analyses.

REFERENCES

Braveman, P. 2006. Health disparities and health equity: Concepts and measurement. *Annual Review of Public Health* 27:167-194.

Brennan, L., R. Brownson, and P. Hovmand. No date. Evaluation of active living by design: Implementation patterns across communities. *American Journal of Preventive Medicine* [under review].

Homer, J., and G. Hirsch. 2006. System dynamics modeling for public health: Background and opportunities. *American Journal of Public Health* 96:452-458.

Hovmand, P., D. Andersen, E. Rouwette, G. Richardson, K. Rux, and A. Calhoun. 2012. Group model-building "scripts" as a collaborative planning tool. *Systems Research and Behavioral Science* 29(2):179-193.

Israel, B., E. Eng, A. Schulz, E. Parker, and D. Satcher (eds.). 2005. *Methods in community-based participatory research for health*. San Francisco: John Wiley & Sons.

Krieger, J., C. Allen, A. Cheadle, S. Ciske, J. Schier, K. Senturia, and M. Sullivan. 2002. Using community-based participatory research to address social determinants of health: Lessons learned from seattle partners for healthy communities. *Health Education and Behavior* 29(3):361-382.

Lantz, P., E. Viruell-Fuentes, B. Israel, D. Softley, and R. Guzman. 2001. Can communities and academia work together on public health research? Evaluation results from a community-based participatory research partnership in Detroit. *Journal of Urban Health* 78(3):495-507.

Lincoln, Y. S., and E. G. Guba. 1985. Establishing trustworthiness. In *Naturalistic inquiry*. Beverly Hills, CA: Sage.

Metzler, M., D. Higgins, C. Beeker, N. Freudenberg, P. Lantz, K. Senturia, and A. Elsinger, E. Uiruell-Fuentes, B. Gheisar, A. Palermo, and D. Softley. 2003. Addressing urban health in Detroit, New York City and Seattle through community-based participatory research partnerships. *American Journal of Public Health* 93(5):803-811.

Morecroft, J. 2002. Resource management under dynamic complexity. In *Systems perspectives on resources, capabilities, and management processes*, edited by J. Morecroft, R. Sanchez, and A. Henne. New York: Pergamon. Pp. 19-40.

Morecroft, J. 2008 (July 20-24). *System dynamics, rbv, and behavioural theories of firm performance: Lessons from people express.* Paper presented at the International Conference of the System Dynamics Society, Athens, Greece.

Morecroft, J., R. Sanchez, and A. Henne. 2002. *Systems perspectives on resources, capabilities, and management processes.* New York: Pergamon.

Schulz, A., E. Parker, B. Israel, A. Allen, M. DeCarlo, and M. Lockett. 2002. Addressing social determinants of health through community-based participatory research: The East Side Village Health Worker Partnership. *Health Education and Behavior* 29(3):326-341.

Vennix, J. 1996. *Group model building: Facilitating team learning using system dynamics.* New York: John Wiley & Sons.

Vennix, J. 1999. Group model building: Tackling messy problems. *System Dynamics Review* 15(4):379-401.

Wallerstein, N. 1999. Power between evaluator and community: Research relationships within New Mexico's healthier communities. *Social Science and Medicine* 49(1):39-53.

Warren, K. 2002. *Competitive strategy dynamics.* New York: Wiley.

C

Open Meeting Agendas

MEETING 1
JUNE 20, 2011

Agenda

10:30–10:45 a.m.	Welcome and Introductions *Robert Lawrence, Chair*
10:45–11:20 a.m.	Sponsor Presentation of Charge
10:45–11:10 a.m.	*The Robert Wood Johnson Foundation* *Angela McGowan*
11:10–11:30 a.m.	*W.K. Kellogg Foundation* *Brian Smedley*
11:30 a.m.–12:00 p.m.	Discussion
12:00 p.m.	**ADJOURN**

MEETING 2
SEPTEMBER 19, 2011

8:30 a.m.	Welcome and Introduction *Robert Lawrence, Chair*

| 8:45–9:15 a.m. | Sponsor Charge
Marion Standish, The California Endowment
James Sprague, Chairman and CEO,
de Beaumont Foundation |

| 9:15–9:30 a.m. | Committee Question and Answer |

Frameworks for Assessing Value

Each presenter will be given 20 minutes to describe the framework used to assess value. Each presenter will be asked to conclude with thoughts of how the framework discussed might be applicable to valuing community-based, non-clinical prevention interventions to improve health.

| 9:30–9:50 a.m. | Framework for Decision Making on Obesity Prevention
Harold Sox
Dartmouth Medical School |

| 9:50–10:10 a.m. | Discussion |

| 10:10–10:30 a.m. | What Works?: Policies and Programs to Improve Wisconsin's Health
Bridget Booske
University of Wisconsin–Madison |

| 10:30–10:50 a.m. | Discussion |

| **10:50-11:10 a.m.** | **BREAK** |

| 11:10–11:30 a.m. | Valuing Housing Subsidies
Robert Haveman
University of Wisconsin–Madison |

| 11:30 a.m.–12:00 p.m. | Discussion |

| **12:00–1:00 p.m.** | **LUNCH** |

| 1:00–1:20 p.m. | Assessing the Impact of the Federal Empowerment Zone Program
Deirdre Oakley
Georgia State University |

1:20–1:40 p.m.   Discussion

Incorporating Assessments of Value into Policy

Each person will have 20 minutes for a presentation about using assessments of value to make policy decisions.

1:40–2:00 p.m.   Impact of Targeted Beverage Taxes
                        Chen Zhen
                        RTI International

2:00–2:20 p.m.   Discussion

2:20–2:40 p.m.   Economics of Early Childhood Policy
                        M. Rebecca Kilburn
                        RAND

2:40–3:00 p.m.   Investment in Early Childhood Development
                        Rob Grunewald
                        The Federal Reserve Bank of Minneapolis

3:00–3:40 p.m.   Discussion

3:40–4:00 p.m.   **BREAK**

4:00–5:00 p.m.   Open Testimony. Individuals who have signed
                        up in advance will be given 3 minutes each to
                        describe what they think should be included in
                        measures to value community-based, non-clinical
                        prevention policies and wellness strategies.

5:00 p.m.   **ADJOURN**

MEETING 3
DECEMBER 5, 2011

8:30–8:45 a.m.   Welcome
                        Robert Lawrence, Committee Chair
                        Professor of Environmental Health
                        *   Sciences, Health Policy, and International*
                        *   Health*
                        Director, Center for a Livable Future
                        Bloomberg School of Public Health

8:45–9:15 a.m.	Framework for Evaluating Health Promotion projects
	Brenda Spencer
	Institute of Social and Preventive Medicine
	University of Lausanne
	Switzerland
9:15–9:45 a.m.	Discussion
9:45–10:15 a.m.	Designing and Evaluating Health Promotion Programs: The PIPE Approach
	Nicolaas Pronk
	Vice President
	Center for Health Promotion
	HealthPartners
10:15–10:45 a.m.	Discussion
10:45–11:00 a.m.	**BREAK**
11:00 a.m.–12:15 p.m.	Issues and Challenges in Assigning Value to Prevention
11:00–11:20 a.m.	*Steven H. Woolf*
	Director, Center for Human Needs
	Virginia Commonwealth University
11:20–11:40 a.m.	*Tyler Norris*
	Chief Executive Officer
	Tyler Norris Associates, Inc.
11:40 a.m.–12:15 p.m.	Discussion
12:15–1:15 p.m.	**LUNCH**
1:15–1:45 p.m.	Weight Loss Program Savings for Medicare
	Kenneth Thorpe
	Chair, Department of Health Policy and Management
	Rollins School of Public Health
	Emory

1:45–2:15 p.m.	Discussion
2:15–2:35 p.m.	Community-Based Program Perspective on Assigning Value *Veva Islas-Hooker* *Regional Program Coordinator* *Central California Regional Obesity* *Prevention Project*
2:35–3:00 p.m.	Discussion
3:00 p.m.	**ADJOURN**

D

Committee Biographical Sketches

Robert S. Lawrence, M.D. (*Chair*), is the Center for a Livable Future Professor and professor of environmental health sciences, health policy, and international health at the Johns Hopkins Bloomberg School of Public Health and professor of medicine at the Johns Hopkins School of Medicine. Dr. Lawrence is a graduate of Harvard College and Harvard Medical School, and trained in internal medicine at the Massachusetts General Hospital in Boston. He served for 3 years as an epidemic intelligence service officer at the Centers for Disease Control and Prevention (CDC), U.S. Public Health Service.

Dr. Lawrence is a master of the American College of Physicians and a fellow of the American College of Preventive Medicine. He is a member of the Institute of Medicine, the Association of Teachers of Preventive Medicine, the American Public Health Association, and Physicians for Human Rights. From 1970 to 1974, he was a member of the faculty of medicine at the University of North Carolina at Chapel Hill, where he helped develop a primary health care system funded by the Office of Economic Opportunity. In 1974, he was appointed the first director of the division of primary care at Harvard Medical School, where he subsequently served as the Charles S. Davidson Associate Professor of Medicine and chief of medicine at the Cambridge Hospital until 1991. From 1991 to 1995, he was the director of health sciences at the Rockefeller Foundation.

From 1984 to 1989, Dr. Lawrence chaired the U.S. Preventive Services Task Force of the Department of Health and Human Services and served on its successor, the Preventive Services Task Force, from 1990 to 1995. He currently serves as a consultant to the Task Force on Community Preventive

Services at the CDC. Dr. Lawrence has participated in human rights investigations on behalf of Physicians for Human Rights and other human rights groups in Chile, Czechoslovakia, Egypt, El Salvador, Guatemala, Kosovo, the Philippines, and South Africa.

In 1996, Dr. Lawrence became the founding director of the Center for a Livable Future at the Bloomberg School of Public Health. The center is an interdisciplinary group of faculty and staff that focuses on equity, health, and the Earth's resources. Research, education, and advocacy examine the relationships among diet, food production systems, the environment, and human health. The center's website is http://www.jhsph.edu/clf.

Kirsten Bibbins-Domingo, Ph.D., M.D., M.A.S., is associate professor of medicine and epidemiology and biostatistics at the University of California, San Francisco (UCSF), an attending physician at San Francisco General Hospital, and the co-director of the UCSF Center for Vulnerable Populations. Dr. Bibbins-Domingo is an active researcher in preventive cardiology, the epidemiology of cardiovascular disease in young adults, and race- and gender-related health and health care disparities. Her research has examined the development of cardiovascular risk factors in young adults, the effectiveness of screening and diagnostic tests for cardiovascular disease, computer-simulated projections of future cardiovascular disease trends, and the impact of public health and clinical interventions on cardiovascular disease prevention. She is an inducted member of the American Society for Clinical Investigation. Dr. Bibbins-Domingo served on the Institute of Medicine (IOM) Committee on Evaluation of the Presumptive Disability Decision-Making Process for Veterans from 2006 to 2007 and the IOM Vaccine Safety Committee from 2010 to 2011. She is currently a member of the U.S. Preventive Services Task Force. Dr. Bibbins-Domingo received her undergraduate degree in molecular biology and public policy from Princeton University and her medical degree, Ph.D. in biochemistry, and master's in clinical research from the UCSF.

Laura K. Brennan, Ph.D., M.P.H., is founder, president, and CEO of Transtria LLC, a certified, woman-owned, small public health research and consulting company in St. Louis, Missouri, with a vision of uniting people, places, and policies to revolutionize public health. She is an assistant professor of behavioral science and health education in the department of community health at Saint Louis University School of Public Health. Dr. Brennan has led multiple projects at the national, state, and local levels with practitioners, researchers, providers, community members, and advocacy groups, related to designing, planning, implementing, or evaluating research- and practice-based efforts to address social, economic, and environmental influences on behaviors and health.

Dr. Brennan has published 19 peer-reviewed articles studying behaviors and health. She is the lead author on *Promoting Healthy Equity: A Resource to Help Communities Address Social Determinants of Health* (a publication of the CDC); a co-author on *Tailoring Health Messages: Customizing Communication with Computer Technology*; and a co-author on *Local Government Actions to Prevent Childhood Obesity* (a publication of the IOM). She is president of the board for the Missouri Family Health Council.

Norman Daniels, Ph.D., is the Mary B. Saltonstall Professor and professor of ethics and population health in the department of global health and population at the Harvard School of Public Health. Formerly chair of the philosophy department at Tufts University, where he taught from 1969 to 2002, his most recent books include *Just Health: Meeting Health Needs Fairly* (2008); *Setting Limits Fairly: Learning to Share Resources for Health*, 2nd edition (2008); *From Chance to Choice: Genetics and Justice* (2000); and *Is Inequality Bad for Our Health?* (2000). His research is on justice and health policy, including priority setting in health systems, fairness and health systems reform, health inequalities, and intergenerational justice. He directs the ethics concentration of the health policy Ph.D., recently won the Everett Mendelsohn Award for mentoring graduate students, and teaches courses on ethics and health inequalities and justice and resource allocation.

Darrell J. Gaskin, Ph.D., researches primarily the determinants of access and quality of health services for minority, Medicaid, uninsured, chronically ill, and other vulnerable populations, disparities in health care, and the hospital safety net. He seeks to understand the role of segregation, market level, and other contextual factors on disparities in health and health services use.

Lawrence W. Green, M.P.H., Dr.P.H., is the co-director of the society, diversity, and disparities program at the UCSF. Before joining the Centers for Disease Control and Prevention as a distinguished fellow/visiting scientist in 1999, Dr. Green was director of the Institute of Health Promotion Research in the faculty of graduate studies and professor of health care and epidemiology in the faculty of medicine at the University of British Columbia, where he also headed the division of preventive medicine and health promotion. Dr. Green received his degrees in public health at the University of California (UC), Berkeley. He worked as a health educator in local, state, and federal health agencies in California and for the Ford Foundation in Dhaka, East Pakistan (now Bangladesh), and served as the first director of the U.S. Office of Health Information and Health Promotion. He has served on the public health faculties at UC Berkeley, Johns Hopkins University, Harvard University, University of Texas, University of British Columbia, and Emory University's Rollins School of Public Health, and now at the UCSF. Dr. Green serves as the Kaiser Family Foundation's vice president and director of its national health promotion program, which received the Foundation Award of the National Association of Prevention Professionals.

Robert Haveman, Ph.D., is the John Bascom Professor of Economics and Public Policy, department of economics and Robert M. La Follette Institute of Public Affairs, and research affiliate, Institute for Research on Poverty at the University of Wisconsin–Madison. He received his B.A. degree from Calvin College in 1958 and his Ph.D. in economics from Vanderbilt University in 1963. Prior to 1970, he was professor of economics at Grinnell College, senior economist at the Joint Economic Committee, U.S. Congress, and research professor at the Brookings Institution. From 1970 to 1975, he was director of the Institute for Research on Poverty. In 1975-1976, Dr. Haveman was a fellow at the Netherlands Institute for Advanced Study, and in 1984-1985 he served as Tinbergen Professor at Erasmus University, The Netherlands. From 1988 to 1991, he was director of the Robert M. LaFollette Institute of Public Affairs, and from 1993 to 1996 served as chair of the department of economics. He was co-editor of the *American Economic Review* from 1985 to 1991. His primary fields of interest are public finance, the economics of poverty, and social policy (including disability policy).

Jennifer Jenson, M.P.H., M.P.P., is a managing senior fellow at Partnership for Prevention. In this role, she leads work to demonstrate the value of clinical and community preventive services, and helps develop and promote the organization's policy agenda. She is committed to developing and applying evidence-based methods to evaluate preventive services, using evidence in policy making, and presenting information in a format that is helpful for decision makers. Before joining Partnership for Prevention, Ms. Jenson spent most of her professional career as a policy advisor to the U.S. Congress. Her experience includes analytic and management roles at the Congressional Budget Office, the Medicare Payment Advisory Commission, and the Congressional Research Service. In addition to these congressional roles, Ms. Jenson has worked on Medicaid policy at the White House Office of Management and Budget. She holds master's degrees in public health and public policy from the University of Michigan and undergraduate degrees in political science and public health from UC San Diego.

F. Javier Nieto, M.D., Ph.D., is chair of the department of population health sciences, Helfaer Professor of Public Health, and professor of population health sciences and family medicine at the University of Wisconsin School of Medicine. His research interests include cardiovascular disease epidemiology, markers of subclinical atherosclerosis, emerging risk factors for cardiovascular disease, and health consequences of sleep disorders and psychosocial stress. He is co-author of a textbook on intermediate epidemiology methods titled *Epidemiology: Beyond the Basics*, and has served as a member of the editorial board of the *American Journal of Epidemiology*. Dr. Nieto received his M.D. from the University of Valencia, Spain, and completed a residency in family and community medicine. After a brief period working for the Spanish government in developing primary health care centers in a rural area of central Spain, he came to the United States. He earned an M.H.S. and Ph.D. in epidemiology at Johns Hopkins University.

Daniel Polsky, Ph.D., is professor of medicine in the division of general internal medicine and professor of health care management in the Wharton School at the University of Pennsylvania, and the director of research at the Leonard Davis Institute of Health Economics. In 2007-2008 he was the senior economist on health issues at the President's Council of Economic Advisers. He received a Ph.D. in economics from the University of Pennsylvania in 1996 and a master's in public policy from the University of Michigan in 1989. He was awarded the Samuel Martin Health Evaluation Sciences Research Award in 2005. His research areas include health insurance and financial access to health care, economic evaluation of medical and behavioral health interventions, and the health care workforce. The link between all of his research is a commitment to establishing causal relationships among either medical or health system interventions and health and economic outcomes using randomized trials, administrative clinical data, and national health surveys. In addition to his publications in the *Journal of Health Economics*, *Health Services Research*, and *Medical Care*, he is a co-author of the book *Economic Evaluation in Clinical Trials*, recently published by Oxford University Press.

Louise Potvin, Ph.D., completed her doctorate in public health and post-doctoral training in program evaluation at the Université de Montréal. She is currently professor in the department of social and preventive medicine, Université de Montréal, and scientific director of the Centre Léa-Roback sur les Inégalités Sociales de Santé de Montréal. She holds the CHSRF/CIHR Chair on Community Approaches and Health Inequalities. This chair aims to document how public health interventions in support of local social development contribute to the reduction of health inequalities in urban settings. Her main research interests are the evaluation of community health promotion programs and how local social environments are conducive to health. She was a member of the World Health Organization (WHO)–Europe Working Group on the Evaluation of Health Promotion. She is a member of the Canadian Reference Group on the Social Determinants of Health and the WHO Scientific Resource Group on Health Equity Analysis and Research. She is a globally elected member of the board of trustees of the International Union for Health Promotion and Education and a fellow of the Canadian Academy of Health Sciences.

Nicolaas P. Pronk, Ph.D., is vice president for health management and health science officer for JourneyWell at HealthPartners in Minneapolis, Minnesota, and senior research investigator at the HealthPartners Research Foundation. Dr. Pronk holds an adjunct faculty position as professor of society, human development, and health at the Harvard School of Public Health. Dr. Pronk is widely published in both the scientific and practice literature and a national and international speaker on health and productivity management. He is president of the International Association for Worksite Health Promotion and a member of the Task Force on Community Preventive Services. Formerly, Dr. Pronk served on the Clinical Obesity Research Panel at the National Institutes of Health, the Carter Center Medical Home initiative, the Defense Health Board (Armed Forces Epidemiological Board), the Health Promotion Advisory Panel at the National Committee for Quality Assurance, and the Institute of Medicine's Committee to Assess Health Promotion Programs at NASA. He is the senior editor of *ACSM's Worksite Health Handbook,* 2nd edition, and the author of the scientific background paper for the U.S. National Physical Activity Plan for Business and Industry. Dr. Pronk received his doctorate in exercise physiology at Texas A&M University and completed his postdoctoral studies in behavioral medicine at the University of Pittsburgh Medical Center and Western Psychiatric Institute and Clinic in Pittsburgh, Pennsylvania.

Louise B. Russell, Ph.D., is research professor at the Institute for Health, Health Care Policy, and Aging Research, and professor in the department of economics, Rutgers University. Her research focuses on the methods and application of cost-effectiveness analysis. Before joining Rutgers, Dr. Russell was a senior fellow at the Brookings Institution in Washington, DC. Elected to membership in the IOM in 1983, she has served on several IOM committees, including the National Cancer Policy Board (2001-2005). Dr. Russell co-chaired the U.S. Public Health Service Panel on Cost-Effectiveness in Health and Medicine, which published recommendations for improving the quality and comparability of cost-effectiveness studies in the book *Cost-Effectiveness in Health and Medicine* (Oxford University Press, 1996) and three articles in the *Journal of the American Medical Association* (October 1996). She was also a member of the first U.S. Preventive Services Task Force (1984-1988). Dr. Russell is an associate editor of the journal *Medical Decision Making* and has published many articles and seven books, including *Is Prevention Better Than Cure?* (Brookings, 1986), and *Technology in Hospitals: Medical Advances and Their Diffusion* (Brookings, 1979).

Steven M. Teutsch, M.D., M.P.H., became the chief science officer, Los Angeles County Public Health, in February 2009, where he will continue his work on evidence-based public health and policy. He had previously been in the Outcomes Research and Management program at Merck (since October 1997), where he was responsible for scientific leadership in developing evidence-based clinical management programs, conducting outcomes research studies, and improving outcomes measurement to enhance quality of care. Prior to joining Merck, Dr. Teutsch was director of the Division of Prevention Research and Analytic Methods (DPRAM) at the CDC, where he was responsible for assessing the effectiveness, safety, and cost-effectiveness of disease and injury prevention strategies. DPRAM developed comparable methodology for studies of the effectiveness and economic impact of prevention programs, provided training in these methods, developed CDC's capacity for conducting necessary studies, and provided technical assistance for conducting economic and decision analysis. The division also evaluated the impact of interventions in urban areas, developed the Guide to Community Preventive Services, and provided support for CDC's analytic methods. He has served as a member of that task force and the U.S. Preventive Services Task Force, which develops the Guide to Clinical Preventive Services, as well as on America's Health Information Community Personalized Health Care Workgroup. He currently chairs the Secretary's Advisory Committee on Genetics Health and Society, and serves on the Evaluation of Genomic Applications in Prevention and Practice Workgroup as well as Institute of Medicine panels. Dr. Teutsch joined CDC in 1977, where he was assigned to the Parasitic Diseases Division and worked extensively on toxoplasmosis. He was then assigned to the kidney donor program and subsequently the kidney disease program. He developed the framework for CDC's diabetes control program. Dr. Teutsch joined the epidemiology program office and became the director of the Division of Surveillance and Epidemiology, where he was responsible for CDC's disease monitoring activities. He became chief of the Prevention Effectiveness Activity in 1992.

Dr. Teutsch was born in Salt Lake City, Utah. He received his undergraduate degree in biochemical sciences at Harvard University in 1970, an M.P.H. in epidemiology from the University of North Carolina School of Public Health in 1973, and his M.D. from Duke University School of Medicine in 1974. He completed his residency training in internal medicine at Pennsylvania State University, Hershey. He was certified by the American Board of Internal Medicine in 1977 and the American Board of Preventive Medicine in 1995, and is a fellow of the American College of Physicians and the American College of Preventive Medicine. Dr. Teutsch is an adjunct professor at the Emory University School of Public Health, Department of Health Policy and Management and the University of North Carolina School of Public Health. Dr. Teutsch has published more than 150 articles and 6 books in a broad range of fields in epidemiology, including parasitic diseases, diabetes, technology assessment, health services research, and surveillance.

Chapin White, Ph.D., is a senior health researcher at the Center for Studying Health System Change (HSC) who has focused on microsimulation modeling of health reform, long-term trends and geographic variation in health spending, medical malpractice, nonprofit hospitals, and Medicare payment policy. At HSC, he is focusing on policy analyses relating to the implementation of health reform and original research quantifying the likely impacts of health reform. Dr. White was formerly a principal analyst at the Congressional Budget Office, a postdoctoral fellow at the National Bureau of Economic Research, a consultant to the Medicare Payment Advisory Commission, and an analyst at Abt Associates. He earned his doctorate in health policy from Harvard University, a master's degree in public policy from Harvard's Kennedy School of Government, and a bachelor's degree in social anthropology, cum laude, from Harvard.